Temporal Bone Imaging

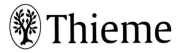

Temporal Bone Imaging

Ellen G. Hoeffner, MD
Associate Professor
Neuroradiology Fellowship Program Director
Department of Radiology
University of Michigan Medical School
Ann Arbor, Michigan

Suresh K. Mukherji, MD
Professor and Chief of Neuroradiology
  and Head and Neck Radiology
Professor of Radiology, Otolaryngology–
  Head and Neck Surgery, and Radiation
  Oncology
University of Michigan Medical School
Ann Arbor, Michigan

Dheeraj Gandhi, MD
Assistant Professor
Department of Radiology
University of Michigan Medical School
Ann Arbor, Michigan

Hemant Parmar, MD
Assistant Professor
Department of Radiology
University of Michigan Medical School
Ann Arbor, Michigan

Diana Gomez-Hassan, MD, PhD
Assistant Professor
Department of Radiology
University of Michigan Medical School
Ann Arbor, Michigan

Vaishali Phalke, MD
Assistant Professor
Department of Diagnostic Radiology
Oregon Health and Science University
Portland, Oregon

Sachin Gujar, MD
Lecturer
Department of Radiology
University of Michigan Medical School
Ann Arbor, Michigan

Douglas J. Quint, MD
Professor of Neuroradiology/MRI
Department of Radiology
University of Michigan Medical School
Ann Arbor, Michigan

Mohannad Ibrahim, MD
Assistant Professor
Department of Radiology
University of Michigan Medical School
Ann Arbor, Michigan

Ashok Srinivasan, MD
Assistant Professor
Department of Radiology
University of Michigan Medical School
Ann Arbor, Michigan

Gaurang V. Shah, MD
Assistant Professor
Department of Radiology
University of Michigan Medical School
Ann Arbor, Michigan

Thieme
New York • Stuttgart

Thieme Medical Publishers, Inc.
333 Seventh Ave.
New York, NY 10001

Editor: Timothy Hiscock
Editorial Assistant: David Price
Vice President, Production and Electronic Publishing: Anne T. Vinnicombe
Production Editor: Print Matters
Vice President, International Marketing and Sales: Cornelia Shulze
Chief Financial Officer: Peter van Woerden
President: Brian D. Scanlan
Compositor: Compset, Inc.
Printer: The Maple-Vail Book Manufacturing Group

Library of Congress Cataloging-in-Publication Data

Temporal bone imaging / Ellen G. Hoeffner ... [et al.].
     p. ; cm.
   Includes bibliographical references and index.
   ISBN 978-1-58890-401-0 (Americas : alk. paper) -- ISBN 978-3-13-140231-8 (rest of world : alk. paper)
     1. Temporal bone--Imaging. 2. Temporal bone--Diseases--Diagnosis. I. Hoeffner, Ellen G.
   [DNLM: 1. Temporal Bone--radiography. 2. Diagnostic Imaging. 3. Ear Diseases--diagnosis. 4. Temporal Bone--pathol-
ogy. WE 705 T2888 2008]
   RF235.T46 2008
   617.8'407572--dc22

                                                                                                    2007044533

Important note: Medical knowledge is ever-changing. As new research and clinical experience broaden our knowledge, changes in treatment and drug therapy may be required. The authors and editors of the material herein have consulted sources believed to be reliable in their efforts to provide information that is complete and in accord with the standards accepted at the time of publication. However, in view of the possibility of human error by the authors, editors, or publisher of the work herein or changes in medical knowledge, neither the authors, editors, or publisher, nor any other party who has been involved in the preparation of this work, warrants that the information contained herein is in every respect accurate or complete, and they are not responsible for any errors or omissions or for the results obtained from use of such information. Readers are encouraged to confirm the information contained herein with other sources. For example, readers are advised to check the product information sheet included in the package of each drug they plan to administer to be certain that the information contained in this publication is accurate and that changes have not been made in the recommended dose or in the contraindications for administration. This recommendation is of particular importance in connection with new or infrequently used drugs.

Some of the product names, patents, and registered designs referred to in this book are in fact registered trademarks or proprietary names even though specific reference to this fact is not always made in the text. Therefore, the appearance of a name without designation as proprietary is not to be construed as a representation by the publisher that it is in the public domain.

Printed in the United States

5 4 3 2 1

ISBN   978-1-58890-401-0

In loving memory of my parents, Alfred and Grace Hoeffner, for their unconditional guidance, support and love. To my husband, Julius, you are everything to me.

Ellen G. Hoeffner

In loving memory of my parents, Chandra Mukherji, MD and Phatick Mukherji, MD, who loved me with all their hearts and taught me that no hard work goes unrewarded. To my wife, Rita Patel, MD, for putting up with me for the past 15 years. And to my children, Anika and Janak, to whom I entrust my heart and our future.

Suresh K. Mukherji

To Bobby, my wife and a true friend. Thanks for helping me at every step of the way. To Shreya, my daughter, for her unconditional love, smiles, and hugs.

Dheeraj Gandhi

To my wonderful children, Alex, Adriana, Nadina and Omar, whom I love very much.

Diana Gomez-Hassan

To my parents, Drs. Krishnakant and Mamata Gujar, and my wife, Bansari, for their support and love through it all.

Sachin Gujar

To my parents, two great people in my life, my loving wife, and all of my family, friends, and teachers, who gave me more than I can give back.

Mohannad Ibrahim

To my parents and all my teachers for guiding me through difficult turns in life. To my wife for her love and support.

Hemant Parmar

To my family, parents, who made it all possible, my husband, Vinayak, and my daughters, Vidisha and Aarushi, for their love and patience. To my teachers and colleagues for all the teaching.

Vaishali Phalke

To my parents, Barbara and George; my sons, Mark and Jason; and my wife, Leslie, for always being there.

Douglas J. Quint

To Prachi and Navya, the delights in my life.

Ashok Srinivasan

To my parents, Vrindavan and Vinu Shah, for their unconditional love and support; Kinnari, for taking the journey with me; and Sharvil and Sahil, for bringing joy into our life.

Gaurang V. Shah

CONTENTS

SECTION IV
Inner Ear and Petrous Bone

PREFACE

Temporal bone imaging is arguably one of the most challenging areas of interpretation for radiologists. The difficulty arises from what we may consider the "perfect storm" of a knowledge gap. First of all, for those of us who are more "mature," our only exposure to the temporal bone anatomy in medical school was schematic illustrations in our anatomy and histology textbooks. We had very little opportunity to directly view the components of the middle and inner ear in gross anatomy compared to other structures of the body such as the liver, leg, or bowel! Secondly, the common pathology involving the temporal bone is unique and was not part of the standard medical school curriculum or clinical rotations. Most of us were only exposed to the clinical disorders if we rotated in an ENT elective during medical school. Lastly, most of us had very little dedicated instruction in the cross-sectional anatomy of the temporal bone on CT or MRI during our radiology training, unless we had faculty who completed a neuroradiology fellowship (rare!) or focused on head and neck imaging (even rarer!!). With this as a backdrop, practicing radiologists are then asked to interpret complex studies in which we lack a fundamental knowledge base. Thus, it is easy to see why most radiologists consider temporal bone imaging very perplexing.

It is with this in mind that we undertook this project in hopes of "demystifying" the temporal bone. This teaching atlas presents the most common temporal bone pathology that you will encounter in your practice. We have divided the text into seven sections (Anatomy, External Auditory Canal, Middle Ear and Mastoid, Inner Ear and Petrous Bone, Trauma, Postoperative Ear, and Miscellaneous). Within each section are chapters devoted to specific disease entities. Each chapter has a standard format that consists of epidemiology, clinical findings, pathology, treatment, and imaging findings. We have tried to be comprehensive but succinct when writing the text of each chapter in order to emphasize the major teaching points. Each chapter has representative illustrations that identify the typical findings that you may encounter in your practice. There are also chapters specifically devoted to the anatomy of the temporal bone and facial nerve.

We feel that this textbook will have a broad appeal. Because of the atlas format, the book will be beneficial for practicing radiologists as a ready reference. The consistent format and succinct summaries should also be helpful for radiology residents and neuroradiology fellows preparing for their board and CAQ examinations. General otolaryngologists and otologists may also find this text useful due to the large number of cross-sectional images of the various disease entities. This was a "labor of love" and we hope you will find our textbook useful in your practice.

Acknowledgment
The authors would like to thank Anne Phillips for her wonderful illustrations for the book.

CHAPTER 1 Temporal Bone
Dheeraj Gandhi

Embryology

The temporal bones contain the sensory organs of hearing and balance, and these are located along the lateral and basal aspect of the skull. Each temporal bone consists of five parts: the squamous, the mastoid, the tympanic, zygomatic, and petrous segment (**Fig. 1–1A**). Important vascular channels, including the carotid artery and jugular vein, course through the temporal bone. The temporal bone is intimately related to the dura of the middle and posterior cranial fossa.

Squamous Portion

The squamous portion is composed of a flat plate of bone that forms the lateral wall of the middle cranial fossa and medial wall of the high masticator space. The outer surface is smooth and convex; it provides attachment to the temporalis muscle. A curved line (the temporal line) runs upward and backward along the posterior part, serving as an attachment for the temporalis fascia. The outer surface also demonstrates a vertical groove for the middle temporal artery. The squamous portion contributes to the posterior segment of the zygomatic arch and forms the anterior, or articular, portion of the mandibular fossa. The mandibular fossa is bounded anteriorly by the articular tubercle and posteriorly by the tympanic part of the temporal bone, which separates it from the external acoustic meatus.

The internal surface of the squamous temporal bone is concave and forms the lateral wall of the middle cranial fossa (**Fig. 1–1B**). It protects the lateral aspect of the temporal lobe of the brain. Branches of the middle meningeal vessels are related to the inner surface. Its superior border is formed by the squamosal suture, where it contacts the parietal bone. The anteroinferior border is thick and serrated; it articulates with the greater wing of the sphenoid.

Tympanic Portion

The tympanic portion is a U-shaped, curved bony plate that forms much of the external auditory canal (EAC) and the posterior (nonarticular) part of the glenoid fossa. It is located below the squamous portion and in front of the mastoid portion. The posterosuperior surface is concave, forming the anterior wall, the floor, and part of the posterior wall of the bony external acoustic meatus. The anteroinferior surface constitutes the posterior boundary of the mandibular fossa, and is related to the retromandibular part of the parotid gland.

The lateral border is free and gives attachment to the cartilaginous part of the external acoustic meatus. The tympanic sulcus is located on its medial aspect, providing the attachment for the tympanic membrane.

Styloid Portion

The styloid process is a thin and pointed bony projection that extends inferiorly from the posterolateral aspect of the inferior surface of the petrous bone. The proximal part is ensheathed by the vaginal process of the tympanic portion and it is located at the anterior margin of the stylomastoid foramen.

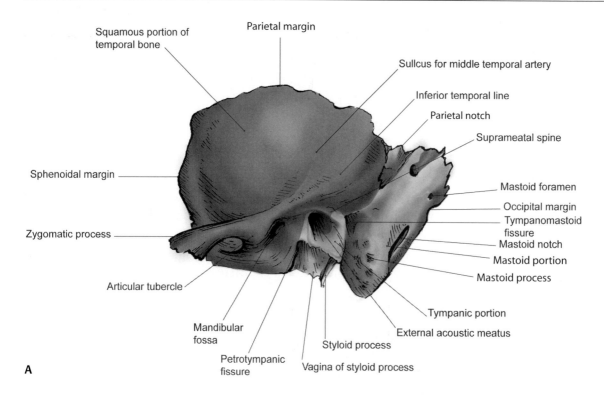

A

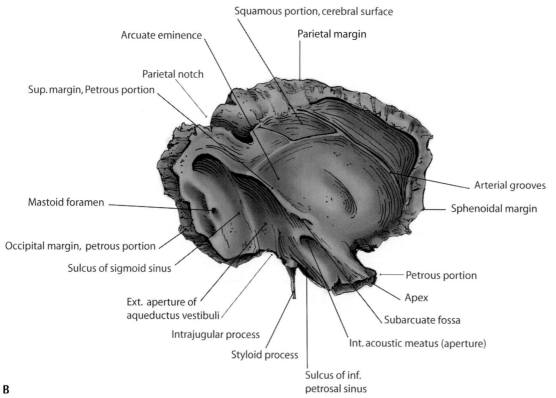

B

Figure 1–1 Labeled schematic illustrations of the **(A)** lateral and **(B)** medial surface anatomy of the temporal bone. (See Color Plate 1–1A,B)

Its distal part gives attachment to the stylohyoid and stylomandibular ligaments. In addition, the styloglossus, stylohyoideus, and stylopharyngeus muscles also have their origins from the distal part of the styloid process. The stylohyoid ligament extends from the apex of the process to the lesser cornu of the hyoid bone. It can be partially or completely ossified.

Mastoid Portion

The mastoid is a pneumatized, bulbous, bony process at the most posterior and inferior part of the temporal bone. It is somewhat triangular in shape, with the vertex directed inferiorly and the base superiorly.

Anteriorly, the mastoid process forms the tympanomastoid suture as it joins the posterior portion of the tympanic bone. Above and lateral to the tympanomastoid suture is a variably sized suprameatal spine, an osseous elevation that anchors the nonosseous portion of the auricle to the EAC.

The mastoid articulates with the parietal bone superiorly and the occipital bone inferiorly, forming the parietomastoid and the occipitomastoid sutures. These two sutures join the occipitoparietal suture at a point called the asterion, an important surgical landmark for posterior fossa craniotomies.

On the medial side of the mastoid tip is a deep groove, the mastoid notch, for the attachment of the digastric muscle, running from anterior to posterior. At its anterior termination, the sulcus serves as a landmark for the descending portion of the facial nerve and the stylomastoid foramen.

The inner surface of the mastoid portion bears a curved groove, the sigmoid sulcus, which lodges part of the transverse sinus. This groove for the transverse sinus is separated from the innermost of the mastoid air cells by a very thin lamina of bone.

The size of the mastoid is a reflection of its extent of the pneumatization. The degree of pneumatization can be extensive or minimal, depending on the genetic influences and presence of chronic infection during development. The air cells usually extend from the mastoid antrum to the mastoid tip, and occupy the retrofacial area and the perilabyrinthine region. The mastoid antrum is the largest and most constant air cell, located at the upper and front part of the bone. It opens anteriorly into the portion of the tympanic cavity that is known as the attic or epitympanic recess. The roof of the antrum is formed by a thin plate of bone called the tegmen mastoideum that separates it from the middle cranial fossa.

Petrous Portion

The petrous bone is a pyramid-shaped wedge of bone that forms the most medial aspect of the temporal bone. The petrous apex is directed medial, forward, and slightly cranial. Viewed from above and from inside the cranium, the base of the pyramid is the lateral surface that articulates with the squamous, tympanic, and mastoid portions of the temporal bone. The three sides of the pyramid are the superior surface that constitutes much of the floor of the middle cranial fossa, a medial surface that faces the posterior cranial fossa, and the inferior surface that articulates with the occipital bone posteriorly.

The superior surface forms an important part of the middle cranial fossa floor. At its most anterior portion is the foramen lacerum, through which the internal carotid artery passes at the end of its horizontal portion. Near its junction with the greater wing of the sphenoid is the foramen ovale where the third division of the trigeminal nerve (cranial nerve [CN] V$_3$) exits the skull base entering the infratemporal fossa. The foramen spinosum is lateral and posterior to the foramen ovale and transmits the middle meningeal artery. A small impression of the superior semicircular canal, the arcuate eminence, can be usually seen along the superior surface. It is usually, but not always, elevated above the surrounding bone, the lateral portion of which forms the tegmen mastoideum and the tegmen tympani.

The medial or cerebellar surface of the temporal bone forms the anterolateral wall of the posterior fossa. Near its center is a large orifice, the internal acoustic meatus (porus acusticus). It leads into a short canal, approximately 1 cm in length, which runs laterally. It transmits CNs VII and VIII. The meatus ends laterally at the medial wall of the vestibule and the inferior surface of the modiolus and basal cochlear turn. A horizontal bony ridge (crista falciformis) located at the lateral limit divides the meatus into two compartments, superior and inferior. The upper compartment is also divided into anterior and posterior portions by a small vertical bony crest commonly known as Bill's bar. These bony ridges divide the fundus of the internal auditory canal (IAC) into four quadrants, each carrying its own cranial nerve: the anterior-superior with the facial nerve, the anterior-inferior with the cochlear, and the posterior-superior and posterior-inferior quadrants occupied by the superior and inferior vestibular nerves, respectively.

The inferior surface is irregular, and forms part of the undersurface of the base of the skull. The inferior surface articulates with the occipital bone forming the petro-occipital suture almost in continuity to the occipitomastoid suture. The jugular foramen is located here with its lateral margin formed by the petrous bone and its medial margin by the occipital bone. Immediately anterior to the jugular foramen is the petro-occipital sulcus, which contains the inferior petrosal sinus. In addition to the internal jugular vein, CNs IX, X, and XI also exit the cranial cavity by the jugular foramen. The cranial nerves are separated from the venous components by a dural septum and fibrovascular tissue. Lateral and anterior to the anterior component of jugular foramen is the ascending portion of the carotid canal at the petrous portion's junction with the tympanic bone.

The petrous bone houses the middle and inner ear structures. Detailed description of these cavities and structures is available in Chapters 3 and 5.

Suggested Readings

Curtin HD, Sanelli PC, Som P. Temporal bone: Embryology and Anatomy. In: Som P, Curtin HD, ed. Head and Neck Imaging, 4th ed. St. Louis: Mosby, 2003:1057–1092

Donaldson JA, Duckert LG, Lambert PM, Rubel EW. Surgical Anatomy of the Temporal Bone, 4th ed. New York: Raven Press, 1992:19–31

Gray's Anatomy, 38th ed. New York: Churchill Livingstone, 1995:1367–1397

Smark A. Anatomy and diseases of the temporal bone. In: Atlas SW, ed. Magnetic Resonance Imaging of the Brain and Spine, 2nd ed. Philadelphia: Lippincott-Raven, 1996:998–999

Embryology

The external auditory canal (EAC) is a derivative of first branchial cleft that lies between the first (mandibular) and second (hyoid) branchial arches. The first branchial cleft or groove is derived from ectoderm and contributes to form the EAC, the cuticular layer of the tympanic membrane, and the tympanic ring. During embryogenesis, the dorsal portion of the first branchial cleft persists to form the EAC, whereas the ventral portion disappears. However, persistence of the ventral portion may result in the development of a first branchial cleft anomaly, for example a cyst, sinus, or fistula.

Although the ectoderm of the medial first branchial cleft begins to invaginate around the 4th week of embryonic development, the corresponding endodermal evagination from the pharynx grows outward and the two come in contact briefly. The first pharyngeal pouch subsequently becomes the eustachian tube, the tympanic cavity, and its epithelial lining. By the 5th week of embryonic development, mesoderm grows between the ectodermal and endodermal layers, and ultimately the tympanic membrane is formed by all three germinal layers.

Ectoderm of the first branchial cleft gives rise to the EAC, which develops as an invagination at the site of the future auricle at the 4th gestational week. By the 8th week, a solid core of epithelium arises and extends to the area of the middle ear space, separated from it by a thin layer of mesoderm. At approximately 28 weeks, this core begins to recanalize from medial to lateral until the surface ectoderm is reached, giving rise to the external auditory canal. At its medial extent, ectoderm persists as the outermost layer of the tympanic membrane, with the mesodermal layer reduced to a fibrous sheet interposed between outer ectoderm and inner cuboidal endoderm.

The auricle develops around the first branchial groove from six focal outgrowths (hillocks of His) arising from the first and second branchial arches. These hillocks fuse by the 3rd month of intrauterine life. The tympanic membrane, ossicles, and otic capsule are generally fully developed at birth, but the EAC undergoes further developmental changes after birth through approximately 9 years of age. In neonates, the EAC is almost straight and the floor of the bony canal is only partially ossified. The bony canal undergoes complete ossification by age 3 or 4. Defective ossification of the anteroinferior EAC may result in a persistent defect (foramen of Huschke). By about age 9, the EAC has a fully developed S-shaped configuration. In adults, the tympanic membrane subtends approximately 45 degrees from the horizontal.

Anatomy

The EAC consists of a lateral fibrocartilaginous portion and medial bony canal (**Fig. 2–1A,B**). The junction of the cartilaginous and the bony portions is the narrowest portion of the EAC and it is called the "isthmus." The lateral, cartilaginous portion of the EAC is oriented in a posterosuperior direction, and the medial, bony portion of the canal is oriented in an anteroinferior direction. Therefore, pulling the pinna outward, upward, and backward aligns the lateral and medial portions of the canal in a straight line and permits visualization of the tympanic membrane.

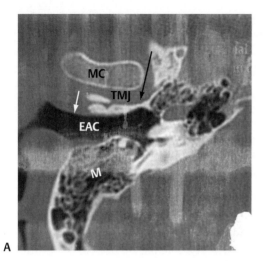
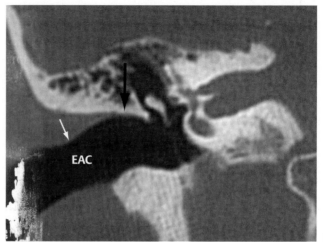

Figure 2–1 **(A)** Axial and **(B)** coronal computed tomograph of the external auditory canal (EAC): membranous po of EAC (*small arrow*), and bony portion of EAC (*large arr w*).

TMJ, temporomandibular joint; MC, mandibular condyle; M, mastoid air cell.

There are two to three vertically oriented deficiencies (Santorini fissures) in the anteroinferior aspect of the cartilaginous canal. These Santorini fissures can serve as conduits for possible extension of infection from the EAC to the parotid space. The medial two thirds of the EAC is composed of bone and consists of a tunnel though the temporal bone.

The lower part of the posterior wall, the floor and the anterior wall, are formed by the tympanic portion of the temporal bone. The roof and the remainder of the posterior wall arise from the squamous temporal bone. The EAC is lined by keratinizing stratified squamous epithelium. The skin of the bony canal is continuous with the epithelial lining of the lateral aspect of the tympanic membrane. In the medial aspect of the EAC, the skin lacks the adnexal structures and subcutaneous layer. Here, the skin is adherent to the periosteum of the bone. However, the skin of the cartilaginous canal is thicker, contains a well-developed subcutaneous layer, and bears the hair follicles and numerous sebaceous and ceruminous glands.

The blood supply to the medial EAC comes mainly from the deep auricular branch of the internal maxillary artery. The lateral EAC is mainly supplied by the branches of posterior auricular and superficial temporal arteries. Venous drainage is mainly via posterior auricular and superficial temporal veins, which subsequently drain into the external jugular, internal jugular, or mastoid emissary veins. Lymphatics typically follow the veins and drain to parotid, postauricular lymph nodes as well as superficial cervical nodes.

The cutaneous innervation of the EAC is complex, with cranial nerves (CNs) V, VII, IX, and X providing contributions. The auricle also receives a portion of its sensory innervation from the cervical plexus via the great auricular nerve. The auriculotemporal branch of the mandibular division of CN V supplies the superior and anterior aspects of the canal and the anterior portion of the tympanic membrane. The posterior and inferior aspects of the canal are supplied by CNs VII, IX, and X via the auricular branch of the vagus (Arnold nerve). Arnold nerve receives contributions from CNs VII and IX as it traverses the temporal bone and then exits the bone via the tympanomastoid suture or stylomastoid foramen. This complex innervation mediates clinical phenomena of referred otalgia from other head and neck structures and the initiation of coughing during manipulation of the ear canal.

Suggested Readings

Donaldson JA, Duckert LG, Lambert PM, Rubel EW. Surgical Anatomy of the Temporal Bone, 4th ed. New York: Raven Press, 1992:19–31

Gray's Anatomy, 38th ed. New York: Churchill Livingstone, 1995:1367–1397

Moore KL. The Developing Human: Clinically Oriented Embryology, 4th ed. Philadelphia: WB Saunders, 1988:402–420

Remley KB, Swartz JD, Harnsberger HR. The external auditory canal. In: Swartz JD, Harnsberger HR, eds. Imaging of the Temporal Bone, 3rd ed. New York: Thieme, 1998

Embryology

Pharyngeal pouches develop between the branchial arches (the first pouch is found between the first and second branchial arches) in very early embryonic life. The endoderm of the pharyngeal pouches and the ectoderm of the branchial grooves contact each other to form the branchial membranes separating the pharyngeal pouches and the branchial grooves. The epithelium of the first branchial groove briefly touches the endoderm of the first pharyngeal pouch at the site of future tympanic membrane.

The first pharyngeal pouch expands to form a tubotympanic recess. This tubotympanic recess gives rise to the tympanic cavity, the mastoid antrum, and their epithelial lining. Connection between the tubotympanic recess and the pharynx elongates to form the auditory tube. The middle ear ossicles are derived from the first and the second branchial arches. The first branchial arch contributes to bodies of malleus and incus and the second arch forms the crura of the stapes, the lenticular process and long process of the incus, and the manubrium of the malleus.

Anatomy of the Middle Ear

The middle ear is an irregular, air-filled space within the temporal bone. It communicates with the nasopharynx through the auditory tube. It contains a chain of movable bones, which connect its lateral to its medial wall, and serve to convey the vibrations communicated to the tympanic membrane across the cavity to the internal ear. The middle ear can be divided into three parts (**Fig. 3–1**): the mesotympanum or the tympanic cavity proper that lies opposite the tympanic membrane; the epitympanum (or the attic) that lies cranial to the tympanic membrane; and the hypotympanum that forms a variable inferior extension of the middle ear cavity below the level of the tympanic membrane.

The tympanic membrane (TM) consists of three layers. The outer layer is continuous with the squamous epithelium of the external auditory canal (EAC). The central layer consists of fibrous connective tissue and is derived from the mesoderm. The inner mucous membrane is continuous with the lining of the inner ear. The circumference of the TM is thickened and forms a fibrocartilaginous ring that is fixed to the tympanic sulcus at the inner end of the EAC. This sulcus is deficient superiorly at the notch

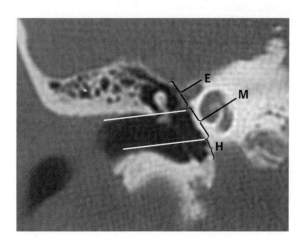

Figure 3–1 Coronal localizer that helps define the location of the epitympanum (E), mesotympanum (M), and hypotympanum (H).

8

of Rivinus. Two bands, the anterior and posterior malleolar folds, take origin from the edges of the notch of Rivinus and extend inferiorly to the lateral process of the malleus. The smaller, triangular part of the TM situated above these folds is lax and thin, and is termed pars flaccida. The manubrium of the malleus is firmly attached to the medial surface of the membrane at a depression called the umbo. The remaining TM is taut and is referred to as the pars tensa. The Prussak space is an important space that is delineated laterally by the pars flaccida, superiorly by that lateral malleolar ligament, inferiorly by the short process of malleus, and medially by the malleolar neck. The epitympanum is bounded laterally by the scutum, derived from the squamous portion of the temporal bone (**Fig. 3–2**).

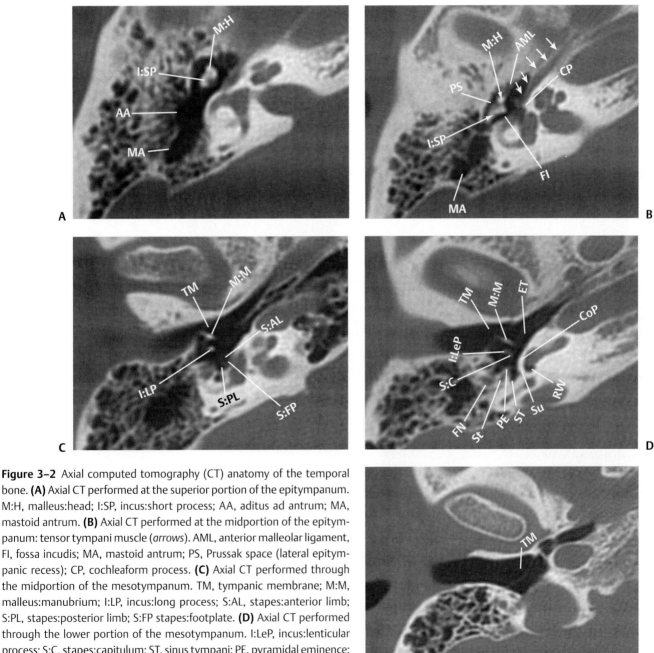

Figure 3–2 Axial computed tomography (CT) anatomy of the temporal bone. **(A)** Axial CT performed at the superior portion of the epitympanum. M:H, malleus:head; I:SP, incus:short process; AA, aditus ad antrum; MA, mastoid antrum. **(B)** Axial CT performed at the midportion of the epitympanum: tensor tympani muscle (*arrows*). AML, anterior malleolar ligament, FI, fossa incudis; MA, mastoid antrum; PS, Prussak space (lateral epitympanic recess); CP, cochleaform process. **(C)** Axial CT performed through the midportion of the mesotympanum. TM, tympanic membrane; M:M, malleus:manubrium; I:LP, incus:long process; S:AL, stapes:anterior limb; S:PL, stapes:posterior limb; S:FP stapes:footplate. **(D)** Axial CT performed through the lower portion of the mesotympanum. I:LeP, incus:lenticular process; S:C, stapes:capitulum; ST, sinus tympani; PE, pyramidal eminence; St, stapedius muscle; FN, descending portion of the facial nerve; Su, subiculum; RW, round window niche; CoP, cochlear promontory; ET, opening of the eustachian tube ("protympanum"). **(E)** Axial CT obtained through the hypotympanum. Note the absence of ossicular structures in the hypotympanum. The main component is air.

The roof of the tympanic cavity is formed by the tegmen tympani. The tegmen tympani separates the epitympanic cavity inferiorly from the middle cranial fossa superiorly. Backward extension of the tegmen forms the roof of the mastoid antrum.

The floor of the tympanic cavity, also referred to as the jugular wall, is a thin plate of bone separating the hypotympanum from the jugular bulb. Many variations can be encountered in the morphology of the jugular bulb, most commonly the asymmetric size of the bulb and the high-riding jugular bulb. The floor of the tympanic cavity may be dehiscent and may permit bulging of the jugular bulb within the tympanic cavity (**Fig. 3–3**).

The anterior (or carotid) wall of the tympanic cavity bears the openings for the eustachian tube and the semicanal for the tensor tympani muscle. The tensor tympani semicanal lies superior to the tympanic orifice of the eustachian tube. The tendon of the tensor tympani makes a right-angle turn at the cochleariform process and attaches to the malleus. The thin plate of cortical bone in the anterior tympanic wall separates it from the carotid canal. This plate is perforated by the tympanic branch of the internal carotid artery and the caroticotympanic nerve.

The medial wall of the middle ear exhibits many important structures. The cochleariform process is located at the level of the junction of the attic and the mesotympanum. The tendon of the tensor

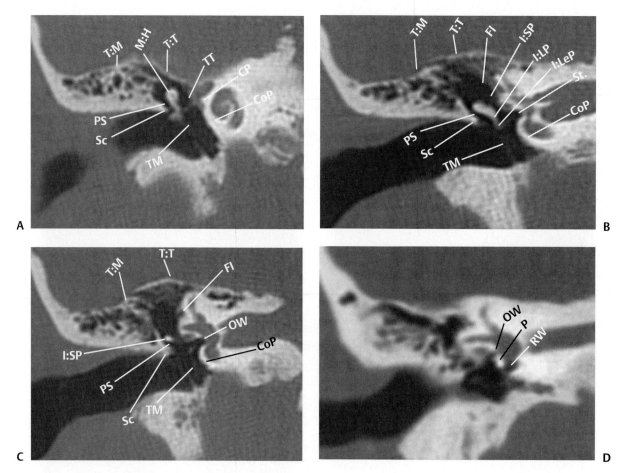

Figure 3–3 Coronal CT anatomy of the temporal bone **(A)** Coronal CT obtained through the midportion of the malleus in the anterior portion of the middle ear cavity. T:T, tegmen tympani; T:M, tegmen:mastoideum; TM, tympanic membrane; PS, Prussak's space (lateral epitympanic recess); Sc, scutum; M:H, malleus:head; TT, tensor tympani; CP, cochleaform process; CoP, cochlear promontory. **(B)** Coronal CT obtained through the midportion of the incus in the midportion of the middle ear cavity. T:T, tegmen tympani; FI, fossa incudis; I: SP, incus:short process; I:LP, incus:long process; I:LeP, incus: lenticular process; St, stapes; CoP, cochlear promontory. **(C)** Coronal CT obtained at the level of oval window.

tympani muscle emerges laterally from this structure to reach the neck of the malleus. Immediately anterior to the cochleariform process is the canal of the tensor tympani muscle, the inferior portion of which is the medial osseous margin of the eustachian tube. The horizontal portion of the facial nerve canal is located just posterior and medial to the cochleariform process, and it contains the tympanic segment of the facial nerve (CN VII). The promontory is a rounded prominence, formed by the projection bulge of the first turn of the cochlea. At the posterosuperior portion of the promontory, just inferior to the facial nerve canal, is the oval window niche that contains the stapes crura and footplate. At the posterior aspect of the promontory, inferior to the oval window, is the round window niche. This niche contains the round window, which is covered by the secondary tympanic membrane.

The posterior wall of the tympanic cavity is formed by the mastoid bone and has three important landmarks: the sinus tympani, the pyramidal eminence, and the facial nerve recess. The pyramidal eminence lies at the medial aspect of the facial recess anterior to the mastoid portion of the facial nerve. Therefore, the facial recess is located lateral to the pyramidal process and the sinus tympani medial to it. The facial nerve recess is the shallower depression and marks the location of the bony canal of descending facial nerve. The tendon of the stapedius muscle emerges from the pyramidal eminence and attaches to the stapes and its neck between the head and the posterior crus. The superior aspect of the posterior wall of mesotympanum communicates with the mastoid through an opening called the aditus ad antrum.

The ossicular chain is composed of three bones: the malleus, the incus, and the stapes. The malleus is the most lateral ossicle and consists of a head, neck, handle or manubrium, and umbo. The head is located in the epitympanum or attic, articulating with the body of the incus. Prussak space separates the malleus head from the lateral bony wall of the attic and is also important in the genesis of secondary cholesteatoma. At the lower and lateral part of the neck of the malleus is the short or anterior process. The tendon of the tensor tympani muscle attaches to the neck just inferior and medial to the short process.

The incus is in the middle and consists of a body, short and long processes, and a lenticular process. The short process is directed posteriorly from the body and nestles in the fossa incudis at the lower part of the aditus ad antrum. The long process ends in a flattened bony projection, the lenticular process. The lenticular process articulates with the head of the stapes, forming the incudostapedial joint.

The stapes is the most medial ossicle, has a head, two crura (the anterior and the posterior), and a footplate. The footplate is a thin oval osseous structure that is attached by the annular ligament to the margins of the oval window.

The mastoid bone consists of multiple air-filled spaces (see Chapter 1). The largest air-filled space is the mastoid antrum, communicating with the middle ear via the aditus ad antrum. The facial nerve canal traverses the mastoid bone in a vertical course, just deep to the facial nerve recess. The mastoid air cells usually extend from the antrum to the mastoid tip, and occupy the retrofacial and the perilabyrinthine region. Pneumatization may sometimes extend into the petrous apex and the squamous bone. The mastoid antrum is the largest and most constant air cell. It sometimes has a thin plate of bone parallel to its surface in its anterior region, near the posterior entrance to the aditus ad antrum. This bony plate arises from the medial and superior walls and represents a remnant of the petrosquamous suture known as Körner's septum.

Suggested Readings

Brogan M, Chakeres DW. Computed tomography and magnetic resonance imaging of the normal anatomy of the temporal bone. Semin Ultrasound CT MR 1989;10:178–194

Curtin HD, Sanelli PC, Som PM. Temporal bone: embryology and anatomy. In: Som PM, Curtin HD, eds. Head and Neck Imaging, 4th ed. St. Louis: Mosby, 2003:1057–1093

Gray's Anatomy, 38th ed. New York: Churchill Livingstone, 1995:1367–1397

Gunlock MG, Gentry LR. Anatomy of the temporal bone. Neuroimaging Clin North Am 1998;8:195–209

Moore KL. The Developing Human: Clinically Oriented Embryology, 4th ed. Philadelphia: WB Saunders, 1988:402–420

Swartz JD, Harnsberger HR. Imaging of the Temporal Bone, 2nd ed. New York: Thieme, 1992

Embryology

The facial nerve is the nerve of the second branchial arch. It serves motor as well as sensory functions. It supplies the striated musculature of the face, neck, and stapedius muscle of the middle ear; parasympathetic fibers to the lacrimal, submandibular, and sublingual glands; the seromucinous glands of the nasal cavity; and it conveys taste sensations from the anterior two thirds of the tongue, the palate, and the tonsillar fossae. It also has a small cutaneous sensory component.

After its origin in the medulla, the facial nerve proceeds forward and laterally in the posterior fossa into the internal auditory meatus, in conjunction with the nervus intermedius (sensory component of the facial nerve) and the acoustic nerve. The intracranial segment of the facial nerve is 23 to 24 mm in length. On entering the internal auditory canal (IAC), the facial nerve occupies the anterosuperior quadrant of this canal for 8 to 10 mm. The internal auditory segment is 7 to 8 mm in length and lies superior to the cochlear nerve, passing above the crista falciformis. While within the canal, the motor root is initially separated from the acoustic bundle by the nervus intermedius, and the two roots unite together in the canal to form the combined trunk.

The labyrinthine segment (**Fig. 4–1**) of the facial nerve measures 3 to 4 mm and represents the narrowest portion of the facial nerve. The facial nerve enters the fallopian canal at the fundus of the IAC and extends from the IAC to the geniculate ganglion. When the nerve reaches a point just lateral and superior to the cochlea, it angles sharply forward, nearly at right angles to the long axis of the petrous temporal, to reach the geniculate ganglion. At the ganglion, the direction of the nerve reverses itself, executing a hairpin bend so that it runs posteriorly. This is the first genu of the facial nerve (**Fig. 4–2**). The greater superficial petrosal nerve arises from the geniculate ganglion and supplies parasympathetic fibers to the lacrimal gland and seromucinous glands of the nasal cavity (**Fig. 4–3**).

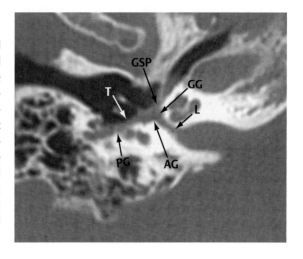

Figure 4–1 The curved reformation of the course of facial nerve nicely demonstrates the various segments of the facial nerve in a single image. The correlative magnetic resonance (MR) scans in the following figures were performed in a patient with Bell palsy that is causing greater than expected enhancement of the facial nerve. However, the enhancement nicely demonstrates the expected location of the nerve in regions of the temporal bone that are often difficult to visualize due to the susceptibility artifact of the surrounding air and adjacent lateral semicircular canal. L, labyrinthine segment; AG, anterior genu; T, tympanic segment; PG, posterior genu; GG, geniculate ganglion; GSP, greater superficial petrosal nerve.

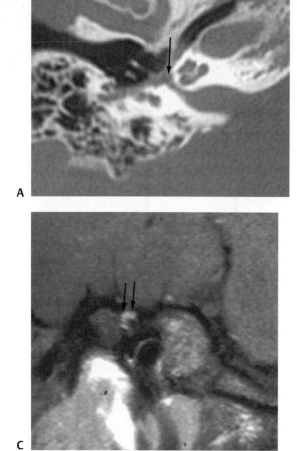

A

B

C

Figure 4–2 (A) Curved reformation of the facial nerve will be used as a localizer for the coronal images through the anterior genu and geniculate ganglion (*arrow*). **(B)** Coronal computed tomography (CT) and **(C)** contrast-enhanced fat-suppressed MR obtained at similar levels through the area of the anterior genu and geniculate ganglion shows the normal location of the nerve at this level (*arrows*).

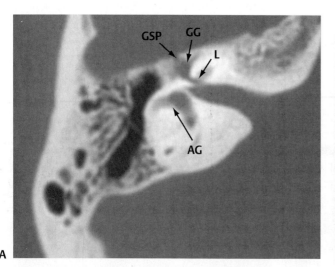

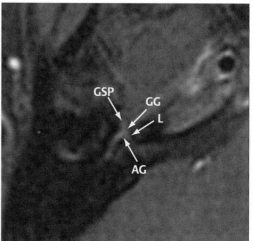

A

B

Figure 4–3 (A) Axial CT and **(B)** contrast-enhanced fat-suppressed MR obtained at similar levels through the epitympanum shows the segmental anatomy of the anterior aspect of the facial nerve. L, labyrinthine segment; AG, anterior genu; GG, geniculate ganglion; GSP, greater superficial petrosal nerve.

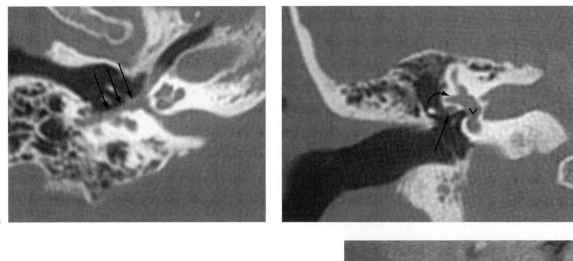

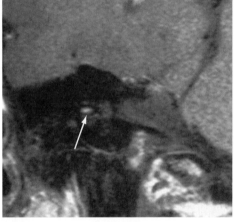

Figure 4–4 Curved reformation of the facial nerve **(A)** will be used as a localizer for the coronal images through the tympanic segment (*arrows*). Coronal CT **(B)** and contrast-enhanced fat-suppressed MR **(C)** obtained at similar levels shows the location of the facial nerve (*arrow*) in the tympanic segment. Lateral semicircular canal (*curved arrow*). V, vestibule.

The tympanic segment (12.0 mm) extends from the geniculate ganglion to the second genu of the facial nerve. It passes posteriorly and laterally along the medial wall of the tympanic cavity (**Fig. 4–4**), perpendicular to the long axis of the petrous bone. Here it lies above the oval window and below the bulge of the lateral semicircular canal (**Fig. 4–5**). At the level of the sinus tympani, the nerve changes direction at the second genu. The mastoid segment (15 to 20 mm) extends from the second genu to the stylomastoid foramen (**Fig. 4–6**). Here the nerve assumes a vertical position, descending in the

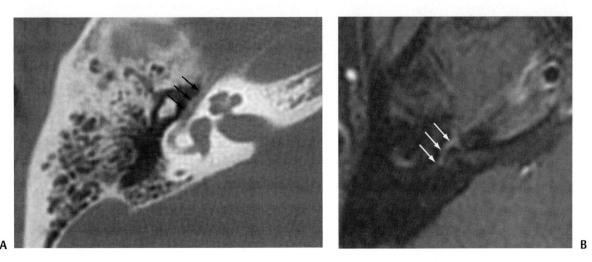

Figure 4–5 **(A)** Axial CT and **(B)** contrast-enhanced fat-suppressed MR obtained at similar levels through the mesotympanum demonstrates the course of the tympanic segment of the facial nerve (*arrows*).

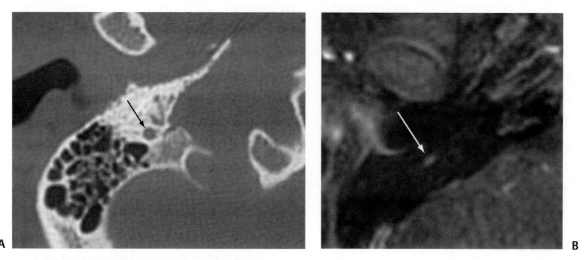

A

B

Figure 4–6 (A) Axial CT and **(B)** contrast-enhanced fat-suppressed MR obtained at similar levels through the mastoid bone shows the descending portion of the facial nerve (*arrow*).

posterior wall of the tympanic cavity and the anterior wall of the mastoid to exit at the base of the skull from the stylomastoid foramen (**Fig. 4–7**). The nerve to the stapedius muscle is a small twig given off from the facial nerve as it descends in the posterior wall of the tympanic cavity behind the pyramidal eminence.

The chorda tympani originates approximately 5 mm above the stylomastoid foramen and carries mostly sensory fibers along with a few parasympathetic fibers. The chorda tympani enters the temporal

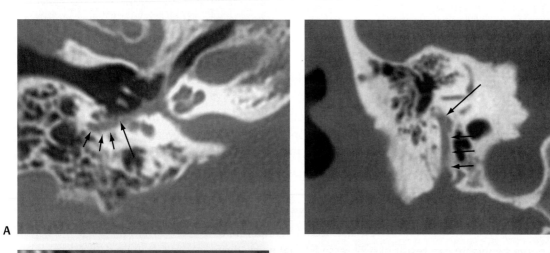

A

B

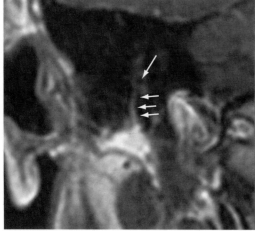

C

Figure 4–7 (A) Curved reformation of the facial nerve will be used as a localizer for the coronal images through the posterior genu (*large arrow*) and descending portion (*small arrows*). **(B)** Coronal CT and **(C)** contrast-enhanced fat-suppressed MR obtained at similar levels through the area of the posterior genu (*large arrow*) and descending portion (*small arrows*) of the facial nerve show the appearance of the expected course of the nerve at this level (*arrows*).

bone as part of the facial nerve; separates laterally from the facial nerve approximately 5 mm superior to the stylomastoid foramen; ascends superiorly in a separate canal to the posterior wall of the middle ear space, and enters the middle ear space via the posterior iter. It enters the tympanic cavity close to the tympanic membrane and crosses the cavity, running along the medial surface of the tympanic membrane. It runs between the malleus and the incus, above the tensor tympani tendon. The chorda exits the temporal bone via the anterior iter in close proximity to the petrotympanic suture and joins the lingual nerve inferior to the skull. This nerve carries taste sensations from the anterior two thirds of the tongue and preganglionic parasympathetic fibers to the submandibular ganglion. This ganglion innervates the submandibular and sublingual salivary glands.

The facial nerve exits from the stylomastoid foramen, crosses lateral to the styloid process, and penetrates the parotid gland. The nerve lies in a fibrous plane that separates the deep and superficial lobes of the parotid gland. In the parotid gland, the nerve divides at the pes anserinus into two major divisions, the superiorly directed temporofacial and the inferiorly directed cervicofacial branches.

After the main point of division, five major branches of the facial nerve exist: temporal (or frontal), zygomatic, buccal, marginal mandibular, and cervical. The facial nerve innervates 14 of the 17 paired muscle groups of the face. The three muscles innervated from other sources include the buccinator, levator anguli oris, and mentalis muscles. Axial and coronal high-resolution computed tomography (CT) forms the mainstay for the imaging of the intratemporal facial nerve, and it can demonstrate exquisite details of entire facial nerve course within the temporal bone. However, CT can only demonstrate the facial nerve canal. Magnetic resonance (MR) can provide direct visualization of the facial nerve itself. The cisternal and internal auditory canal (IAC) segment can be best visualized on submillimetric T2-weighted (T2W) gradient echo or fact spin echo sequences. The intratemporal segment can be investigated with high-resolution postcontrast T1W three-dimensional (3D) gradient echo sequences. On postcontrast T1W images, it is not uncommon to see enhancement of portions of normal facial nerves. This enhancement is most commonly located in the geniculate ganglion, the proximal greater superficial petrosal nerve, and the tympanic segment. This enhancement pattern corresponds to the topography of the circumneural facial arteriovenous plexus and should not necessarily be considered a sign of anatomic abnormality.

Clinical Features

There are many causes of peripheral facial nerve dysfunction. Nearly 80% of facial nerve paralysis is idiopathic (Bell palsy). This is a presumed viral illness that generally resolves spontaneously within 8 weeks. A host of other disorders may also involve the facial nerve. Involvement of the seventh and eighth nerves by herpes zoster can produce sudden hearing loss and facial nerve paralysis (Ramsay Hunt syndrome). Facial nerve may also be damaged by temporal bone fractures.

Facial nerve neoplasm can result in progressive facial nerve dysfunction. The most common tumor to involve the facial nerve is a schwannoma. This tumor has a predilection for involving the geniculate ganglion. Other masses causing facial nerve paralysis in the temporal bone include cavernous hemangiomas, epidermoid cysts, hamartomas, metastases, and perineural extension of parotid malignancies. Lesions at the level of IAC affect facial muscles, taste, lacrimation, the stapedial reflex, and sometimes hearing and balance due to the involvement of cranial nerve VIII.

Suprastapedial lesions located between the nerve to the stapedius and the geniculate ganglion affect facial muscles, taste, and the stapedial reflex, but have no effect on lacrimation, whereas infrastapedial lesions above the chorda tympani branch spare the stapedial reflex too. Infrachordal lesions cause facial paralysis but spare taste, lacrimation, and the stapedial reflex.

Frequent connections between the buccal and zygomatic branches exist. The temporal and marginal mandibular branches are at highest risk during surgical procedures and are usually terminal connections without anastomotic connections. The facial nerve can occasionally be absent congenitally. Portions of the facial nerve canal may demonstrate bony dehiscences. Such dehiscences in the facial nerve canal are most common in the tympanic portion near the oval window and occasionally in the mastoid segment and near the geniculate ganglion.

PEARLS _____

- High-resolution CT of the temporal bone provides detailed anatomy of the bony facial canal in the temporal bone. High-resolution T2W sequences are best in demonstrating the cisternal and IAC segments of the facial nerve. The intratemporal segment can be investigated with high-resolution postcontrast T1W 3D gradient echo sequences.
- Portions of facial nerves may demonstrate enhancement even in normal individuals. Enhancement is most commonly located in the geniculate ganglion, the proximal greater superficial petrosal nerve, and the tympanic segment. However, only enhancement of the labyrinthine segment and the IAC segment is always abnormal.
- Nearly 80% of facial nerve paralysis is idiopathic (Bell palsy), presumably caused by a viral illness. MR can show enhancement of various portions of facial nerve. The nerve is generally not enlarged.
- Schwannoma is the most common primary neoplasm of the facial nerve. It has a predilection for the geniculate ganglion, although it can occur anywhere along the facial nerve course.

Suggested Readings

Chandra S, Goyal M, Gandhi D, Gera S, Berry M. Anatomy of the facial nerve in the temporal bone—HRCT. Indian J Radiol Imaging 1999;9:5–8

Curtin HD, Sanelli PC, Som P. Temporal bone: embryology and anatomy. In: Som P, Curtin HD, eds. Head and Neck Imaging, 4th ed. St. Louis: Mosby, 2003:1057–1092

Ge XX, Spector GJ. Labyrinthine segment and geniculate ganglion of the facial nerve in fetal and adult temporal bones. Ann Otol Rhinol Laryngol Suppl 1981;90:1–12

Gebarski SS, Telian SA, Niparko JK. Enhancement along the normal facial nerve in the facial canal: MR imaging and anatomic correlation. Radiology 1992;183:391–394

Smark A. Anatomy and diseases of the temporal bone. In: Atlas SW, ed. Magnetic Resonance Imaging of the Brain and Spine, 2nd ed. Philadelphia: Lippincott-Raven, 1996:998–999

CHAPTER 5 Inner Ear

Dheeraj Gandhi

Embryology

The maturation of the inner ear involves three main phases:

1. Development (4th to 8th week)
2. Growth (8th to 16th week)
3. Ossification (16th to 24th week)

The development of the sensory epithelium within the membranous labyrinth occurs simultaneously with growth and ossification (8th to 24th week). The inner ear arises from a plate-like thickening of the surface neuroectoderm located between the first branchial groove and the hindbrain, the "otic placode." Each otic placode then invaginates and sinks below the surface neuroectoderm into the underlying mesenchyme, resulting in formation of the "otic pit." The edges of the otic pit fuse to form the otic vesicle (otocyst). The otic vesicle is the precursor of the membranous (or endolymphatic) labyrinth.

When the embryo is 6 to 7 mm in length, the otic vesicle divides into a larger utricular portion and the smaller endolymphatic portion. The dorsally located utricular portion later forms the utricle, semicircular canals, and endolymphatic duct. The ventral saccular portion differentiates into the saccule and the cochlear duct. The primordial cochlear pouch, which develops as an evagination of the saccule, starts to elongate and begins to coil. By the end of the 8th week, the entire membranous labyrinth is identifiable, and formation of the 2½ to 2¾ cochlear turns is complete. The fetus is able to hear with maturation of the organ of Corti, which occurs by the 24th week of gestation (**Fig. 5–1**).

The development of membranous labyrinth is completed by the third trimester. Maturation of sensory end organs occurs first in the utricle and saccule, followed by the semicircular canals and, finally, the cochlea. The cochlea is the last part of the membranous labyrinth to undergo maturation and is therefore more subject to developmental malformations compared with vestibular system. Once the membranous labyrinth has matured (6 to 7 months of fetal age), no further growth occurs during the remaining lifetime of the individual. The only exception is the endolymphatic duct and sac, which continue to grow and reach their mature size after puberty.

The otic capsule is the precursor to the bony labyrinth. The otic capsule develops as a cartilaginous condensation of mesenchyme around the otic vesicle between the 4th and 8th weeks of gestation. Growth of the otic capsule continues to the 16th gestational week. During its growth, vacuoles begin to arise in the cartilaginous otic capsule. These vacuoles eventually coalesce to form the perilymphatic space. The newly created perilymphatic space contains perilymph fluid, which surrounds and bathes the membranous labyrinth. Ossification of the otic capsule occurs between weeks 16 and 24 via 14 ossification centers. The end result is the "bony labyrinth."

Otic capsule ossification is unique in that there are a large number of ossification centers—14—considering the small size of the final product; there is no epiphyseal growth (centers fused directly); and maturation is arrested in a primary state of ossification, that is, endochondral bone persists.

Figure 5–1 Schematic illustration of the anatomy of the cochlea and organ of Corti. (See Color Plate 5–1)

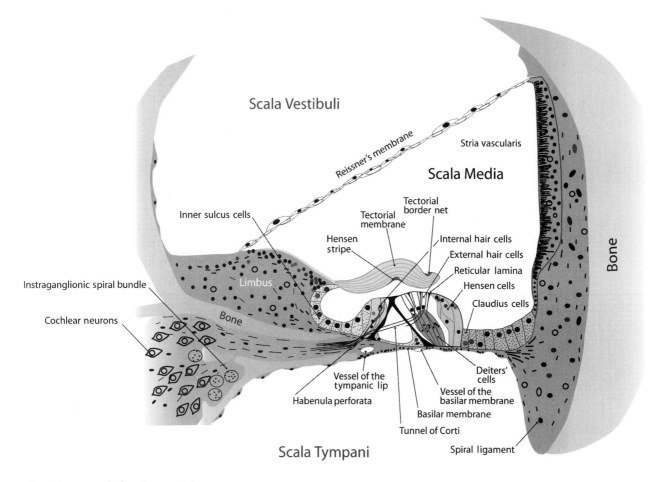

Anatomy of the Inner Ear

The inner ear labyrinth consists of bony and membranous components. The membranous labyrinth contains endolymphatic fluid and it serves as an organ of hearing and balance. The membranous labyrinth is suspended in perilymphatic fluid, which in turn is encased by the bony labyrinth. The bony labyrinth can be divided into three components: the vestibule, the semicircular canals, and the cochlea (**Fig. 5–2**).

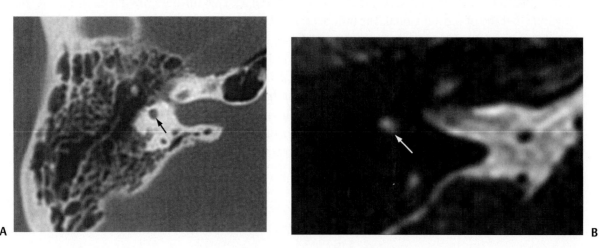

Figure 5–2 (A) Axial computed tomography (CT) and **(B)** T2-driven (T2 DRIVE) equilibrium pulse sequence image through the superior aspect of the epitympanum demonstrates the crux of the superior semicircular canal (*arrows*).

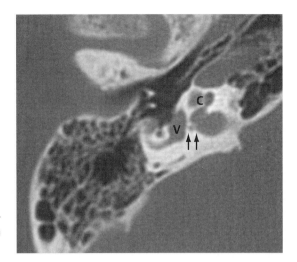

Figure 5–3 Axial CT through the epitympanum obtained inferior to **Figure 5–2**, demonstrating the vestibule (V), cochlea (C), and canal for the superior vestibular nerve (*arrows*).

The Vestibule

The vestibule is a central ovoid cavity within the bony labyrinth, located lateral to the fundus of the internal auditory canal. The vestibule plays a vital role in static balance and is innervated by branches from the vestibular nerve along its medial wall and the floor. The vestibule houses the saccular and utricular portions of the membranous labyrinth and displays a high T2 signal within the signal void of the temporal bone on the magnetic resonance (MR) imaging. The vestibule communicates anteriorly with the cochlea and posteriorly with the semicircular canals (**Fig. 5–3** and **Fig. 5–4**).

The Cochlea

The ability to hear is truly an amazing phenomenon. Hearing arises from the capability to transform mechanical energy to electrical energy. The external ear collects and directs the sound waves to the tympanic membrane. The middle ear converts mechanical motion arising from the tympanic membrane pulsations and transmits it to the fluid in the vestibule via the lever effect of the ossicular chain. The inner ear, specifically the cochlea, transforms fluid motion into electrical energy (**Fig. 5–5**).

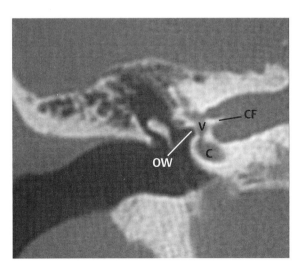

Figure 5–4 Coronal CT obtained through the incus. V, vestibule; C, cochlea; CF, crista falciformis; OW, oval window.

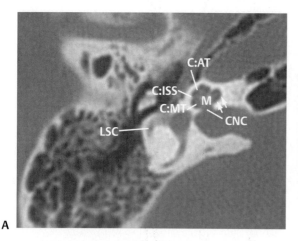

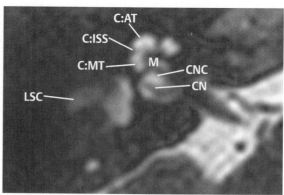

A

B

Figure 5–5 (A) Axial CT and **(B)** T2 DRIVE image obtained inferior to **Figure 5–3**. Osseous spiral lamina (*arrows*). C:AT, cochlea:apical turn; C:ISS, cochlea:interscalar septum; C:MT, cochlea:middle turn; M, modiolus; CN, cochlear nerve; CNC, cochlear nerve canal; LSC, lateral semicircular canal.

The cochlea is a coiled structure consisting of 2½ to 2¾ turns. If it were elongated, the cochlea would be approximately 30 to 32 mm in length. The bony component of the cochlea contains a central bony axis (modiolus), through which the cochlear nerve travels. Projecting outward from the modiolus throughout its length, similar to the head of a screw, is a thin bony plate referred to as the osseous spiral lamina.

The fluid-filled spaces of the membranous cochlea are composed of three parallel canals that are contained with the bony shell of the cochlea: an outer anterior scala vestibuli (ascending spiral) and inner posterior scala tympani (descending spiral) surround the central cochlear duct (scala media). The scala vestibuli and scala tympani contain perilymph and the scala media contains endolymph.

The cochlear duct is separated from the scala vestibuli by the vestibular (Reissner) membrane and from the scala tympani by the basilar membrane. The organ of Corti resides within the cochlear duct on the basilar membrane. The tectorial membrane is adherent to the roof of the organ of Corti, interposed between this structure and the endolymph.

Episodic movement of the stapes results in direct transmission of fluid waves via the oval window through the vestibule and subsequently to the cochlear recess, which lies on the medial wall of the vestibule (**Fig. 5–6** and **Fig. 5–7**). The cochlear recess communicates directly with the scala vestibuli.

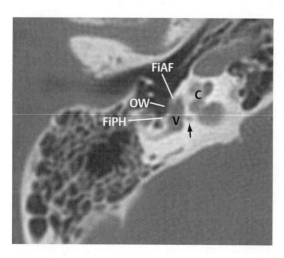

Figure 5–6 Axial CT obtained through the midportion of the middle ear cavity. Singular canal (*arrow*). V, vestibule; C, cochlea; OW, oval window; FoAF, fossula ante fenestram; FiPF, fossula post fenestram.

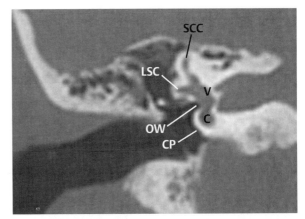

Figure 5–7 Coronal CT obtained posterior to Figure 5–4. V, vestibule; C, cochlea; LSC, lateral semicircular canal; SCC, superior semicircular canal; CP, cochlear promontory; OW, oval window.

Hence, the sounds waves are transmitted directly to the perilymph of the cochlea as fluid waves. These fluid waves are transmitted through the Reissner membrane into the endolymph of the cochlear duct. This causes displacement of the basilar membrane, which stimulates the hair cell receptors of the organ of Corti. It is the movement of these hair cells that generates the electronic potentials that are eventually converted into action potentials in the auditory nerve fibers. It is interesting that the entire fluid volume of the perilymphatic spaces of the inner ear is only 0.2 cc, yet without it hearing would not be possible. The perilymphatic waves are transmitted via the apex of the cochlea from the scala vestibuli (helicotrema) to the scala tympani and eventually dissipated at the round window, which has a flexible diaphragm (**Fig. 5–8** and **Fig. 5–9**).

The basilar membrane varies in width and tension from base to apex. Hence different portions of the membrane respond to different auditory frequencies: higher frequencies closer to the base, lower frequencies closer to the apex. Sensorineural hearing loss may be categorized as sensory (cochlear) loss and neural (retrocochlear) loss. Retrocochlear hearing loss implies involvement of either the cochlear nerve or the cochlear nuclei. Defective function of the cochlea results in sensory (cochlear) loss.

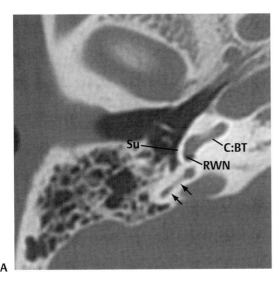

A

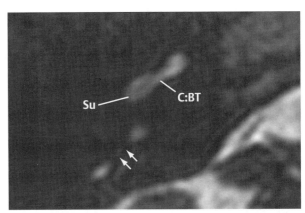

B

Figure 5–8 (A) Axial CT and **(B)** T2 DRIVE obtained through the middle ear cavity inferior to Figure 5–6. Posterior semicircular canal (*arrows*). C:BT, cochlea:basal turn; RWN: round window niche; Su, subiculum.

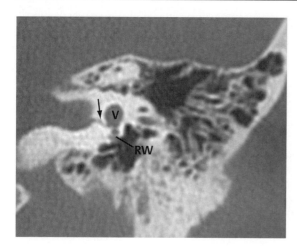

Figure 5–9 Coronal CT obtained posterior to Figure 5–7. Singular canal (*arrow*). V, vestibule; RW, round window.

Vestibular Aqueduct and Endolymphatic Duct System

Vestibular Aqueduct

The vestibular aqueduct (VA) is a bony channel originating from the posterosuperior portion of the vestibule in the vicinity of the common crus. It courses posteriorly, laterally, and inferiorly along the posterior petrous surface. The vestibular aqueduct widens as it approaches its external aperture at the posterior margin of the petrous apex. In the first 20 weeks of fetal life, the course of the VA is straight and parallel to the common crus. As the posterior fossa begins accelerated growth in the final 20 weeks of gestation, the VA and the contents assume its adult J-shaped configuration. The length of the VA is determined by the degree of adjacent pneumatization but is generally approximately 6 to 12 mm in length. Segments of the normal VA are consistently seen with CT imaging. Multiplanar reformations using volume acquisition CT may also be helpful in identifying the complete course of the vestibular aqueduct.

Endolymphatic Duct System

The VA houses the endolymphatic duct (ELD). The anatomy of the endolymphatic apparatus was initially described by Cotugno in 1774. Bast and Anson introduced the term *endolymphatic duct system* (EDS) to refer to the various parts of the endolymphatic duct and sac. The EDS is divided into an endolymphatic sac (ELS) and endolymphatic duct (ELD).

The ELD arises from the union of the utricular and saccular ducts and courses within the bony vestibular aqueduct. As a result, the ELD contains endolymph and is bathed in perilymph. The ELD is also surrounded by loose connective tissue that is continuous with the adjacent periosteum. The ELD can be further divided into two distinct sections: the sinus and isthmus. The sinus (vestibular, horizontal) portion of the ELD is the proximal segment of the ELD, which communicates directly with the saccular and utricular ducts. This narrow, elongated channel terminates where the ELD enters the vestibular aqueduct. The isthmic (vertical) portion is the continuation of the sinus portion and represents the intraosseous segment of the ELD. Histologically, the lining epithelium of the ELD is similar to the utricular and saccular ducts and is composed of simple squamous or low cuboidal cells.

The ELS is the terminal enlargement of the ELD and consists of proximal (rugose) and distal segments. The rugose portion of the ELS is continuous with the distal ELD and consists of a complex network of interdigitating canaliculi and crypts. The proximal rugose portion of the ELS lies within the foveate impression, which is situated along the posterior aspect of the petrous bone and is partially covered by a scale of bone, the operculum. The rugose portion of the ELS has a highly differentiated epithelium consisting of tall cylindrical cells irregularly dispersed into papillae and crypts. The distal segment of the ELS is situated between the periosteal portion of the dura and the dura proper. The distal portion of ELS is lined by cuboidal epithelium.

The arterial supply of the ELS and ELD originates from a dural branch of the stylomastoid artery, which may arise from either the occipital or posterior auricular arteries with equal incidence. The supplying vessels are divided into a superficial component, which directly enter the canaliculi of the vestibular aqueduct and supply the ELS and ELD, and a deep component, which supplies the periductal connective tissue.

The endolymphatic sac and duct are dynamic structures, which have several functions. Recent studies suggest that the cells lining the ELD can alter their shape and size and appear to play a role in the autoregulation of the inner ear ion and fluid balance. Additionally, the presence of cellular debris, macrophages, and a variety of blood cells (predominantly leukocytes) in the lumen of the EDS suggests that the EDS also plays an active role in the immune system of the inner ear.

Suggested Readings

Curtin HD, Sanelli PC, Som PM. Temporal bone embryology and anatomy. In: Som, PM, Curtin HD, eds. Head and Neck Imaging, vol 3, 4th ed. New York: Mosby, 2003:1057–1092

Gadre AK, Fayad JN, O'Leary MJ, Linthicum FH. Arterial supply of the human endolymphatic duct and sac. Otolaryngol Head Neck Surg 1993;108:141–148

Gray's Anatomy, 38th ed. New York: Churchill Livingstone, 1995:1367–1397

Kenna MA. Embryology and developmental anatomy of the ear. In: Bluestone CD, Stool SE, Scheetz MD, eds. Pediatric Otolaryngology, vol 1. Philadelphia: Saunders, 1990:77–87

Lundquist PG, Kimura R, Wersall J. Ultrastructural organization of the epithelial lining in the endolymphatic duct and sac in the guinea pig. Acta Otolaryngol 1964;57:65–80

Mukherji SK, Baggett HC, Alley J, Carrasco VH. Enlarged cochlear aqueduct. AJNR Am J Neuroradiol 1998;19:330–332

Streeter GL. The development of the scala tympani, scala vestibuli and perioticular system in the human embryo. Am J Anat 1917;21:299–320

Streeter GL. The histogenesis and growth of the otic capsule and its contained periotic tissue spaces in the human embryo. Contrib Embryol 1918;20:5–55

Swartz JD, Harnsberger HR. The otic capsule and otodystrophies. In: Swartz JD, Harnsberger HR, eds. Imaging of the Temporal Bone, 2nd ed. New York: Thieme, 1992:192–247

Zechner G, Altman F. Histological studies on the human endolymphatic duct and sac. Pract Otorhinolaryngol (Basel) 1969;31:65–83

Sachin Gujar

Epidemiology

External auditory canal (EAC) dysplasia includes malformations of the external ear (pinna) and EAC. Because the development of the external and middle ear are closely linked, significant malformations of the EAC are usually associated with middle ear abnormalities. Due to the differences in development, inner ear anomalies are less commonly associated, though they are more frequent than in the general population. Congenital aural dysplasia (CAD) is estimated to occur in 1 in 3300 to 1 in 10,000 births and is often an isolated anomaly without a known cause. CAD is unilateral in 70% of cases and is slightly more common in males than females (60% versus 40%). When unilateral, the right ear is more commonly affected than the left. The majority of cases are sporadic, although 14% of cases are familial. CAD can also be associated with genetic disorders, chromosomal aberrations, intrauterine infections, and teratogens.

Embryology

Congenital aural dysplasia results from anomalous development of the first branchial groove. The first branchial groove deepens in the eighth week of gestation to form the lateral third of the EAC. The medial two thirds of the EAC develop from the meatal plate, which is a solid cord of epithelial cells extending from the lateral third of the EAC to the precursor of the middle ear cavity (pharyngeal pouch endoderm). Normally, the meatal plate begins to canalize between the 21st and 26th weeks of gestation. Failure of canalization of the meatal plate results in congenital aural atresia (CAA). Because the first and second branchial pouches and first pharyngeal pouches develop simultaneously, CAA is often associated with anomalies of the middle ear and mastoid.

Clinical Features

Discovery of CAA in a newborn is a cause of great anxiety for the parents, especially when associated with cutaneous manifestations. Patients with CAA are diagnosed early in life and present with a deformity of the auricle and no visible auditory canal. The majority of cases of CAA are sporadic; however, CAA has been associated with various disorders, including Treacher Collins syndrome, Crouzon disease, Klippel-Feil syndrome, Möbius syndrome, Duane syndrome, VATER (vertebral defects, imperforate anus, tracheoesophageal fistula, and radial and renal dysplasia) association, CHARGE (coloboma of the eye, heart anomaly, choanal atresia, retardation, and genital and ear anomalies) association, and Pierre Robin syndrome. Association with a systemic malformation is generally a negative prognostic indicator for successful corrective surgery.

Historically, CAA has been divided into membranous and bony forms. Schuknecht has classified CAA into four types based on a combination of clinical evaluation, surgical findings, and type of repair. Type A is a high-grade meatal stenosis that is limited to the cartilaginous portion of the EAC. Type B is a partial atresia of both the cartilaginous and bony portions of the EAC. This form of CAA is often associated with a short or curved malleus, which may be fixed to the tympanic annulus or wall of the epitympanum. A bony septum may separate the middle ear cavity into a lateral compartment containing the malleus and incus and a medial compartment containing a normal stapes. Type C consists of a completely atretic canal with a well-pneumatized tympanic cavity. There is an atresia plate that may be partial or complete. Characteristically, the malleus and incus are fused; however, the stapes is mobile. The tympanic membrane is absent. The course of the facial nerve is abnormal. In type C atresias, the course of the facial nerve is more anterior and occasionally may overlap the oval window and descend within the atretic plate. Type D is complete atresia with markedly reduced pneumatization of the temporal bone. This form of CAA is associated with anomalies of the bony labyrinth and abnormal course of the facial nerve.

Treatment

Surgical correction of CAA is the treatment of choice, with the form of atresioplasty depending on the type of CAA. In general, surgical correction and imaging is deferred for several years to allow for the development of the temporal bone structures and mastoid. Bilateral EAC atresia is treated early, with the auricular reconstruction preceding atresioplasty. Surgical treatment of unilateral atresia may often be postponed indefinitely, though the cosmetic deformity is treated later in childhood.

Imaging Findings

CT

High-resolution, thin-section computed tomography (CT) is the most important test in patients with aural dysplasia. Since the diagnosis is clinical, the role of CT is preoperative evaluation. EAC dysplasia can be classified as incomplete (stenosis) or complete (atresia), and membranous, bony, or mixed. In the membranous type, soft tissue is seen in the region of the tympanic membrane. In the bony type, the bony plate is variable in thickness. The external ear is also deformed, often small, and dysplastic. There is often poor pneumatization of the tympanic cavity and mastoid, the severity of which is a factor that affects access during surgery.

The ossicular abnormalities seen include fusion of the malleus and incus to the attic wall, fusion of the malleus to the atresia plate, fusion of the malleoincudal articulation, and a dysmorphic shape of

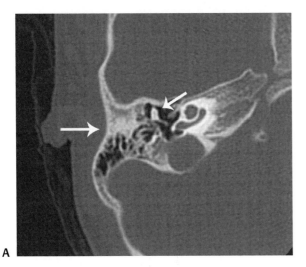
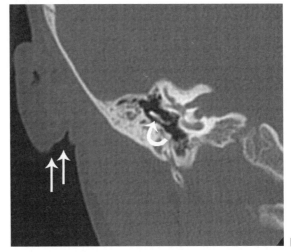

A

B

Figure 6–1 External auditory canal atresia. **(A)** Axial and **(B)** coronal computed tomographic images illustrate lack of the resorption of the embryonic meatal plate (*long arrow*), resulting in a complete bony external auditory canal atresia. The os-sicles are malformed with fusion of the head of the malleus and short process of the incus (*short arrow*). The long process of the incus is also malformed (*curved arrow*). Note the micro-tia of the maldeveloped pinna (*double arrow*).

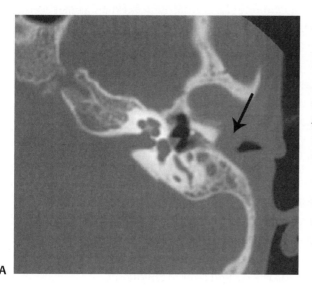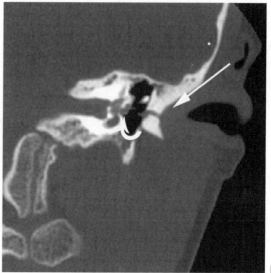

A   B

Figure 6–2 Severe external auditory canal stenosis. **(A)** Axial and **(B)** coronal images CT demonstrate severe stenosis of the external auditory canal. The dysplastic canal (*arrow*) is filled with soft tissue. Abnormal soft tissue is present in the peristapedial region an oval window (*curved arrow*), possibly representing an early cholesteatoma.

the malleus and incus. There can be abnormalities of the oval and round window. Identification of the stapes is very important to the surgeon. Similarly, evaluation of the otic capsule is important since a concurrent inner ear abnormality could preclude surgical treatment.

The course of the facial nerve is almost always abnormal. With the poor development of the tympanic bone, the tympanic segment is often displaced caudally, and the posterior genu and the descending mastoid segment of the facial nerve are typically located more anteriorly or anterolaterally (**Fig. 6–1, Fig. 6–2,** and **Fig. 6–3**).

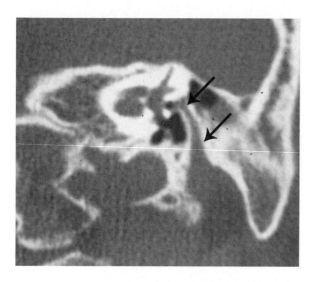

Figure 6–3 Abnormal course of the facial nerve. Coronal CT obtained in a patient with external auditory canal atresia shows an abnormal course of the tympanic and descending segments of the facial nerve (*arrows*).

PEARLS _____

- External auditory canal dysplasia is classified as bony, membranous, or mixed; and incomplete (stenosis) or complete (atresia).
- Associated middle ear deformities include reduced middle ear and mastoid pneumatization, ossicular abnormalities involving the malleus and incus, and a higher incidence of cholesteatomas.
- Identification of a normal inner ear and the presence of stapes are important for surgical planning.
- The course of the tympanic and mastoid segments of the facial nerve is abnormal. The facial nerve usually descends more anteriorly when compared with its normal course.

Suggested Readings

Hudgins PA. EAC atresia. In: Harnsberger HR, ed. Diagnostic Imaging: Head and Neck. Salt Lake City: Amirsys, 2004:I-2–6

Remley KB, Swartz JD, Harnsberger HR. The external auditory canal. In: Swartz JD, Harnsberger HR, eds. Imaging of the Temporal Bone, 3rd ed. New York: Thieme, 1997:16–46

Romo LV, Casselman JW, Robson CD. Temporal bone: congenital anomalies. In: Som PM, Curtin HD, eds. Head and Neck Imaging, 4th ed. St. Louis: Mosby, 2003:1109–1172

Schuknecht HF. Congenital aural atresia and congenital middle ear cholesteatoma. In: Nadol JB, Schuknecht HF, eds. Surgery of the Ear and Temporal Bone. New York: Raven Press, 1993:263–274

CHAPTER 7 External Otitis
Sachin Gujar

Epidemiology

Otitis externa is a common disease affecting all age groups and is usually infective in etiology. Though bacterial infections of the skin of the external auditory canal are the commonest cause, fungal infection can also occur (otomycosis). Infections are more prevalent in hot and humid climate conditions, and are often associated with trauma to the skin of the external auditory canal, such as during mechanical removal of cerumen. Swimming is considered a risk factor, hence the term *swimmer's ear*. Malignant (necrotizing) otitis externa is a particularly aggressive form of infection occurring in a select patient population and is responsible for considerable morbidity and mortality.

Clinical Features

Otitis externa can cause a variable amount of pain (otalgia) and discharge (otorrhea), but it seldom causes significant morbidity. Bacterial infections are usually more symptomatic. Depending on the degree of swelling and debris in the external auditory canal, there may be conductive hearing loss. Systemic signs such as fever and (pretragal) lymphadenopathy may be present.

Malignant (necrotizing) otitis externa is a particularly aggressive life-threatening form of infection caused by *Pseudomonas aeruginosa* infection typically in elderly diabetics and individuals with other immunosuppressed states, such as HIV patients or those who have undergone chemotherapy. Clinically, a high index of suspicion in the susceptible patient population is required for diagnosis. Nonspecific granulation tissue may be seen along the inferior wall of the external auditory canal (at the bony–cartilaginous junction) with exquisitely painful otorrhea. Cranial nerve palsies may result in advanced cases.

Pathology

The commonest organisms responsible are *Staphylococcus aureus* and *Pseudomonas aeruginosa*. Fungal infections with *Candida* and *Aspergillus* are less frequently seen. Malignant otitis externa is associated with aggressive osseous destruction of the temporal bone and mastoid. Advanced cases may result in intracranial and infratemporal extension with meningeal and cranial nerve involvement.

Treatment

Noncomplicated otitis externa is typically treated with topical medications and by keeping the ear dry. Persistent infections, infections with extension beyond the external auditory canal, infections associated with result in cellulitis, and immunocompromised individuals require systemic treatment. Malignant otitis externa is treated with intravenous antibiotics and may need surgical debridement.

Imaging Findings

Imaging is typically not performed for noncomplicated otitis externa. Patients with suspected malignant otitis externa are most often imaged with thin-section computed tomography (CT) of the temporal bone, though magnetic resonance (MR) may also be used.

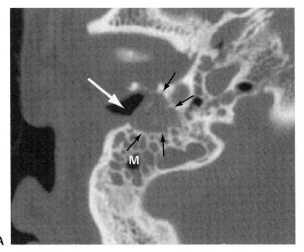

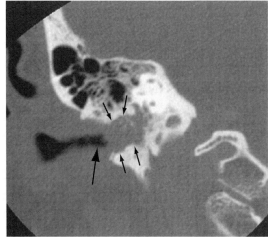

A   B

Figure 7–1 Computed tomography (CT) of malignant otitis externa. **(A)** Axial and **(B)** coronal CT of the right temporal bone reveals an abnormal soft tissue (*large arrow*) mass with destruction of the cortical margins of the external auditory canal (*small arrows*). The internal areas of high attenuation are likely due to adjacent bony destruction. There is opacification of the mastoid air cells (M) identified on the axial images, which may due to direct extension or obstructed secretions.

CT

Bone destruction and invasion of the temporal bone and mastoid are the hallmark of malignant otitis externa. CT is sensitive in detection of early bone erosions. Contrast-enhanced studies are useful in detection of foci of frank pus in the deep facial spaces. Abnormal soft tissue is seen in the external auditory canal and the infratemporal fossa. Facial nerve involvement can occur with infratemporal spread. Other common routes of spread include posterior spread to the mastoid and middle ear, and anteriorly to the temporomandibular joint. Posteromedial spread to the jugular fossa may result in multiple lower cranial nerve palsies. Intracranial spread may result in meningitis, abscess formation, and sigmoid sinus thrombosis. Diffuse skull base osteomyelitis represents an advanced stage of disease (**Fig. 7–1**).

MRI

MRI is superior to CT for the detection of bone marrow edema in skull base involvement and in the evaluation of intracranial complications such as dural, vascular, and cranial nerve involvement (**Fig. 7–2**).

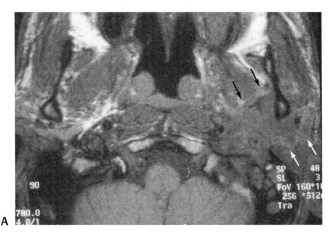

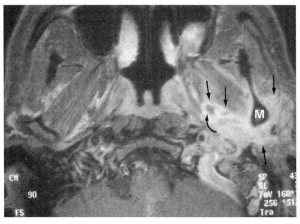

A   B

Figure 7–2 Magnetic resonance (MR) of otitis externa. **(A)** Noncontrast T1-weighted (T1W) image demonstrates a low signal lesion replacing the normal fascial spaces of the lateral masticator space (*arrows*). **(B)** Fat-suppressed postcontrast T1W image shows diffuse enhancement of the inflammatory process, which involves the masticator space (*arrows*) and surrounds the mandible (M). Note the involvement and enlargement of cranial nerve V₃ (*curved arrow*).

Radionuclide Imaging

It has been suggested that anatomic imaging with CT or MR should be supported by routine single photon emission computed tomography (SPECT) bone imaging for initial diagnosis of malignant otitis externa. Technetium-99m (Tc-99m)-methylene diphosphonate (MDP) SPECT imaging, and gallium-67 (Ga-67) scintigraphy or more recently SPECT Indium-111 (In-111) white blood cell (WBC) scanning have been used for the detection and follow-up of disease. Furthermore, these also appear to be the investigations of choice for posttherapeutic assessment.

PEARLS _____

- Imaging is warranted in suspected cases of malignant (necrotizing) otitis externa.
- CT of the temporal bone is the most useful investigation and demonstrates osseous destruction of the temporal bone or the mastoid with enhancing soft tissue in the external ear and adjacent deep neck.
- MR is useful in the evaluation of intracranial complications or nerve involvement.
- CT and MR are excellent in demonstrating the resolution of the soft tissue component but may not be as useful in assessment of the success of osteomyelitis treatment.
- Radionuclide imaging may play a role in the detection of disease and in posttherapeutic assessment of these patients.

Suggested Readings

Davidson HC. Imaging of the temporal bone. Magn Reson Imaging Clin North Am 2002;10:573–613

Harnsberger HR. The temporal bone. In: Harnsberger HR, ed.Handbook of Head and Neck Imaging, 2nd ed. St. Louis: Mosby, 1995:438

Okpala NCE, Siraj QH, Nilssen E, Pringle M. Radiological and radionuclide investigation of malignant otitis externa. J Laryngol Otol 2005;119:71–75

Remley KB, Swartz JD, Harnsberger HR. The external auditory canal. In: Swartz JD, Harnsberger HR, eds. Imaging of the Temporal Bone, 3rd ed. New York: Thieme, 1997:16–46

CHAPTER 8 Cholesteatoma of the External Auditory Canal

Ellen G. Hoeffner

Epidemiology

External auditory canal cholesteatomas (EACC) are rare, with an incidence of 1 in 1000 new otologic patients. Their exact etiology is unknown, and many may occur spontaneously, although prior inflammation, trauma, or surgery have all been associated with EACC. EACC may be caused by loss of normal lateral epithelial migration from the tympanic membrane and external auditory canal (EAC); or increased cellular proliferation induced by accumulation of keratin debris may play a role in the development of these lesions. EAC stenosis or obstruction may also result in EACC. Although EACC can develop in any portion of the canal, the posterior-inferior wall is most common.

Clinical Features

Most patients are adults presenting between 40 and 75 years of age with otorrhea and dull otalgia. Rarely, hearing loss may occur secondary to obstruction of the canal by the EACC. Facial nerve paralysis is even less common. Examination reveals squamous debris protruding from the involved canal wall, which unlike keratosis obturans, does not form a plug. Purulent drainage may be present deeper in the canal due to associated infection. Localized bony erosion is usually present and visible after removal of the debris. Clinically it may appear similar to keratosis obturans, postinflammatory medial canal fibrosis, malignant external otitis, and squamous cell carcinoma.

Pathology

Periostitis of the bony EAC may be the initial abnormality with subsequent invasion by stratified squamous keratinizing epithelium and development of an epithelial lined sac. Release of proteolytic enzymes from the margin of the lesion or secondary bacterial infection resulting in epithelial ulceration and granulation tissue formation may be responsible for bone erosion. Histologically, these lesions consist of stratified squamous keratinizing epithelium sac with periostitis, bone erosion, and sequestration of bone. The tympanic membrane is generally normal.

Treatment

Transaural debridement of the keratin debris and sequestered bone followed by topical antibiotics may be all that is necessary if the entire extent of bone erosion is visualized and symptoms resolve. If conservative therapy is unsuccessful, open debridement, removal of involved bone with a drill, canaloplasty, and split-thickness skin graft may be indicated. Extensive bone loss may necessitate reconstruction with autologous cartilage or bone graft, whereas invasion of mastoid air cells generally requires modified radical mastoidectomy.

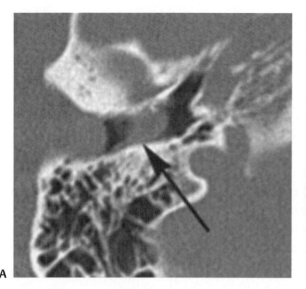
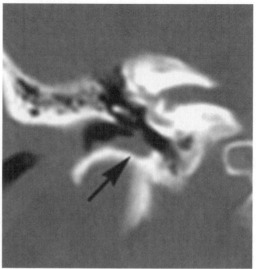

A

B

Figure 8–1 **(A)** Axial computed tomography (CT) of the temporal bone shows a focal mass located in the region of the external auditory canal (*arrow*). The middle ear cavity appears to be well aerated. **(B)** Coronal CT through the tem-poral bone shows the mass to be isolated to the external auditory canal. There is regressive remodeling of the adjacent inferior bony portion of the external auditory canal (*arrow*).

Imaging Findings

CT

Computed tomography (CT) is the imaging modality of choice. EACC is usually seen as a soft tissue attenuation mass in the EAC with adjacent focal bony erosion. The posterior-inferior portions of the canal are most frequently involved, although any portion of the canal can be affected, and there may be circumferential involvement. Small bone fragments can be seen within the soft tissue mass. The lesion may extend into the middle ear or cause erosion of the mastoid air cells, facial nerve canal, or tegmen tympani. Bone erosion associated with EACC may be smooth or irregular. Imaging may show more extensive involvement than was suspected clinically (**Fig. 8–1**).

PEARLS ⎯⎯⎯⎯⎯⎯⎯⎯⎯⎯⎯⎯⎯⎯⎯⎯⎯⎯⎯⎯⎯⎯⎯⎯⎯⎯⎯⎯⎯⎯⎯

- Soft tissue mass in the EAC with adjacent bone erosion, most often along the posteroinferior wall of the canal.
- Sequestra may be seen as small bone fragments within the soft tissue component.
- Assess for extension into the middle ear or erosion of the mastoid air cells, facial nerve canal, and tegmen tympani. Involvement of these structures may change surgical management.

Suggested Readings

Heilbrun ME, Salzman KL, Glastonbury CM, et al. External auditory canal cholesteatoma: clinical and imaging spectrum. AJNR Am J Neuroradiol 2003;24:751–756

Kryzer TC, Lambert PR. Diseases of the external auditory canal. In: Canalis RF, Lambert PR, eds. The Ear: Comprehensive Otology. Philadelphia: Lippincott Williams & Wilkins, 2000:341–357

Martin DW, Selesnick SH, Parisier SC. External auditory canal cholesteatoma with erosion into the mastoid. Otolaryngol Head Neck Surg 1999;121:298–300

Naim R, Linthicum FH. Temporal bone histopathology case of the month: external auditory canal cholesteatoma. Otol Neurotol 2004;25:412–413

Nemzek WR, Swartz JD. Temporal bone: inflammatory disease. In: Som PM, Curtin HD, eds. Head and Neck Imaging, 4th ed. St. Louis: Mosby, 2003:1173–1229

CHAPTER 9 Exostoses

Hemant Parmar

Epidemiology

External auditory canal (EAC) exostoses, also called "surfer's ear" or "cold-water ear," are benign, sessile, multinodular bony masses arising deep in the EAC. They are found commonly in surfers or people with prolonged exposure to cold water. They are known to occur exclusively in humans, and one study found a prevalence rate of 73% in surfers. Prolonged physical, chemical, or thermal irritation is considered the cause of their occurrence.

Clinical Features

The classic age group is young adults, with males affected more than females. The symptoms occur after many years of aquatic exposure. The most common presenting symptom of EAC exostoses is conductive hearing loss. Otitis externa, tinnitus, and otalgia are other symptoms. Most of the cases are bilateral but the presenting symptoms are usually unilateral. Complete occlusion of the canal is rarely seen.

Pathology

External auditory canal exostoses are benign bony overgrowths that show pathologic features similar to osteomas. They also show parallel concentric layers of subperiosteal bone.

Treatment

Asymptomatic exostoses require no active surgical treatment. For patients presenting with conductive hearing loss, resection of these bony overgrowths is undertaken. Other symptoms, such as otitis externa and pain, are managed conservatively.

Imaging Findings

CT

The typically computed tomography (CT) appearance of exostoses is a broad-based, benign-appearing bony protuberance from the osseous portions of the EAC. They show no aggressive features, and the surrounding soft tissue is normal. The most typical appearance is narrowing of the inferior portion of the anterior and posterior walls of EAC. The location is close to the tympanic annulus at the tympanomastoid and tympanosquamous sutures. Intravenous contrast is not required to make the diagnosis (**Fig. 9–1**).

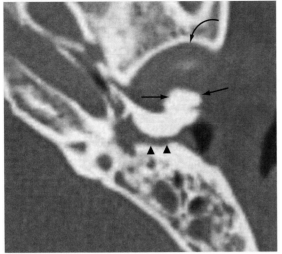
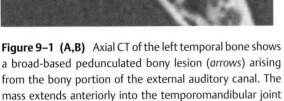

A

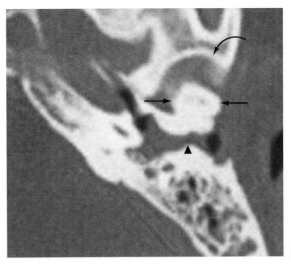

B

Figure 9–1 (A,B) Axial CT of the left temporal bone shows a broad-based pedunculated bony lesion (*arrows*) arising from the bony portion of the external auditory canal. The mass extends anteriorly into the temporomandibular joint (*curved arrow*). The exostosis has resulted in chronic narrowing of the external auditory canal (*arrowheads*). As a result, there is mucosal thickening involving the meatus of the EAC and middle ear cavity.

MRI

Magnetic resonance (MRI) imaging offers no added diagnostic benefit for EAC exostoses. MR imaging shows hypointensity in these masses on both T1- and T2-weighted images. There is no contrast enhancement.

PEARLS _____

- Noncontrast high-resolution CT of the temporal bones with bone algorithm exquisitely delineates these lesions.
- EAC exostoses show bilateral circumferential narrowing of the EAC due to presence of sessile, bony overgrowths from the osseous portions of the EAC.
- MR imaging offers no additional diagnostic benefit.

Suggested Readings

Denia A, Perez F, Canalis RR, Graham MD. Extracanalicular osteomas of the temporal bone. Arch Otolaryngol 1979;105:706–709

Di Bartolomeo JR. Exostosis of the external auditory canal. Ann Otol Rhinol Laryngol 1979;88:2–20

Sheehy JL. Diffuse exostoses and osteomata of the external auditory canal: a report of 100 operations. Otolaryngol Head Neck Surg 1982;90:337–342

Smelt GJ. Exostoses of the internal auditory canal. J Laryngol Otol 1984;98:347–350

CHAPTER 10 External Auditory Canal Osteoma
Ashok Srinivasan

Epidemiology

External auditory canal (EAC) osteomas are rare bony outgrowths found in the EAC and are much less common than EAC exostoses. There is no gender predilection and they may be seen in any age group.

Clinical Features

External auditory canal osteomas are most often asymptomatic and detected incidentally. When they are large, they may cause conductive hearing loss. They can also be associated with serous otitis media and cholesteatoma.

Pathology

Although EAC osteomas commonly reveal a connection to the underlying EAC bone on gross pathologic examination, in some cases there may be no connection demonstrated. They are most commonly seen at the bony–cartilaginous junction of the EAC. On microscopic examination, they are similar to osteomas seen elsewhere and show irregularly oriented lamellated bone surrounding abundant, discrete fibrovascular channels.

Treatment

Since most EAC osteomas are asymptomatic, no treatment is required. In symptomatic patients, supportive medical therapy is often adequate. In select cases, surgical resection under local or general anesthesia provides a permanent cure.

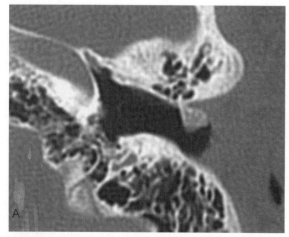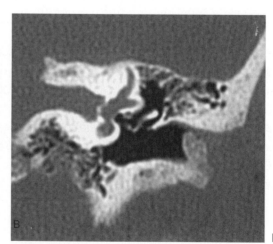

Figure 10–1 (A) Axial and **(B)** coronal noncontrast computed tomography (CT) performed through the left external auditory canal (EAC) shows an EAC osteoma arising from the inferior portion of the EAC at the bony–cartilaginous junction. (Case courtesy of Alexander Arts, MD.)

Imaging Findings

CT

On nonenhanced computed tomography (CT), EAC osteomas are typically solitary bony outgrowths that are pedunculated and unilateral. They are usually small (<1 cm) and are commonly seen at the osseous–cartilaginous junction of the EAC. The overlying soft tissues appear normal and do not reveal any abnormal enhancement (**Fig. 10–1**).

MRI

These lesions are low signal on T1- and T2-weighted images. There is no additional benefit of magnetic resonance (MRI) imaging over CT in EAC osteomas.

PEARLS _____

- Differential diagnosis includes EAC exostosis.
- Although EAC osteoma is pedunculated, solitary, unilateral, and located lateral to the osseous–cartilaginous junction (isthmus), EAC exostoses are usually sessile, bilateral, multilobular, and located medial to the isthmus.

Suggested Readings

Deguine C, Pulec JL. Large osteoma of the external auditory canal. Ear Nose Throat J 2001;80:8

Denia A, Perez F, Canalis RR, Graham MD. Extracanalicular osteomas of the temporal bone. Arch Otolaryngol 1979;105:706–709

Granell J, Puig A, Benito E. Osteoma and exostosis of the external auditory meatus: a clinical diagnosis. Acta Otorrinolaringol Esp 2003;54:229–232

Hsiao SH, Liu TC. Osteoma of the external ear canal. Otol Neurotol 2003;24:960

Kemink JL, Graham MD. Osteomas and exostoses of the external auditory canal—medical and surgical management. J Otolaryngol 1982;11:101–106

Orita Y, Nishizaki K, Fukushima K, et al. Osteoma with cholesteatoma in the external auditory canal. Int J Pediatr Otorhinolaryngol 1998;43:289–293

Pulec JL, Deguine C. Osteoma of the external auditory canal. Ear Nose Throat J 2000;79:908

Ramirez-Camacho R, Vicente J, Garcia Berrocal JR, Ramon y Cajal S. Fibro-osseous lesions of the external auditory canal. Laryngoscope 1999;109:488–491

CHAPTER 11 Squamous Cell Carcinoma
Dheeraj Gandhi

Epidemiology

Tumors of the external auditory canal (EAC) are relatively uncommon. Squamous cell carcinoma represents the most common primary malignant tumor, followed by basal cell carcinoma and adenoid cystic carcinoma. The precise etiology of EAC carcinoma is unknown, but the majority of cases occur in patients with a long history of chronic inflammation of the EAC. Squamous cell carcinoma is encountered more commonly in females, and the median age of occurrence is 55 years.

Clinical Features

The diagnosis and staging of external canal cancer often present a significant challenge. There is usually a long delay that results from the similarity of its presentation with that of more commonly occurring benign inflammatory diseases, such as otitis externa or chronic otitis media, as well as the rarity of the disease. Early diagnosis, which is the single most important prognostic factor, is dependent on a high level of suspicion by the otolaryngologist. Persistent external otitis, despite routine treatment, should increase suspicion of carcinoma and prompt a biopsy. Persistent pain that is out of proportion to clinical abnormality or a change in pain pattern with a chronically painful ear should arouse suspicion. Pain is a common symptom and it often indicates underlying bone involvement. Bloody ear discharge is another hallmark of malignancy, although this is relatively rare. Advanced squamous cell carcinoma can invade adjacent structures, especially the middle ear cleft and parotid gland. Facial weakness may indicate the involvement of cranial nerve VII.

Pathology

External auditory canal carcinomas may appear as polypoidal lesions on clinical inspection. The EAC cartilage does not provide an efficient barrier against tumor spread, and permits radial spread of malignancy. Anteriorly located dehiscences (the fissures of Santorini) and bony–cartilaginous junctions can allow the tumor direct access to the periparotid tissues and temporomandibular joint.

Tumor growth medially along the external ear canal can involve the tympanic membrane and bony tympanic ring, allowing subsequent invasion into the middle ear. Spread into the otic capsule is less common, as dense bone of the otic capsule provides a more effective barrier against tumor spread.

The facial nerve and the stylomastoid foramen serve as metastatic routes to the soft tissues of the neck and the parotid. Proximal extension of malignant cells along the facial nerve (retrograde perineural spread) carries the tumor toward inner ear and posterior fossa.

Nodal metastasis is encountered in advanced malignancies and can be seen in 8 to 10% of cases. The lymphatic drainage of the auricle and EAC extends anteriorly to the periparotid lymph nodes and parotid gland. Drainage to the jugular chain or mastoid group of nodes may also occur.

Treatment

Complete, en-bloc resection of EAC squamous cell carcinomas is the most effective therapy. For lesions confined to the EAC without bone involvement, complete resection may be curative. Radiotherapy often has an adjunctive role in more advanced malignancies. Extension of the tumor into the middle ear cleft reduces 5-year survival from 56% to 27%. Most recurrences tend to be local. Positive surgical margins, despite postoperative radiotherapy, nearly always have a fatal outcome.

Imaging Findings

CT

High-resolution computed tomography (CT), along with a detailed clinical examination can accurately predict the extent of tumor spread and help in staging the disease. Early-stage carcinomas may be seen as areas of nonspecific soft tissue thickening or polypoid mass within the EAC. The mass or area of soft tissue thickening may extend medially into the middle ear. Osseous destruction is easily seen on high-resolution bony algorithm. The tumor can spread anteriorly into the parotid gland or the temporomandibular joint through fissures of Santorini. Posterior extension can be seen into the mastoid air cells. Careful attention should be paid to the facial nerve canal and the stylomastoid foramen. Erosion and asymmetric enlargement of these structures indicate involvement of the facial nerve. Advanced tumors will result in destruction of jugular foramen and the carotid canal and spread into the intracranial cavity (**Fig. 11–1**).

MRI

Although CT scanning forms the mainstay of imaging assessment of EAC carcinomas and demonstration of the extent of bone destruction, magnetic resonance (MRI) may provide complementary evaluation of the soft tissue spread. High-resolution skull base MRI with gadolinium can provide exquisite soft tissue details of the fascial planes and the neurovascular structures. Superior soft tissue resolution and multiplanar nature of MRI can demonstrate parotid and TM joint spread of EAC malignancies that may not be so easily apparent on the CT scan. Similarly, MRI is more sensitive in the assessment of neurovascular structures and intracranial extension of skull base malignancies. Gadolinium-enhanced

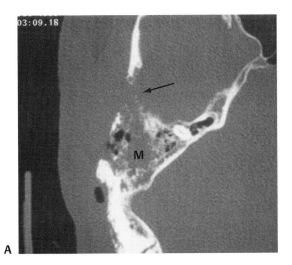

A

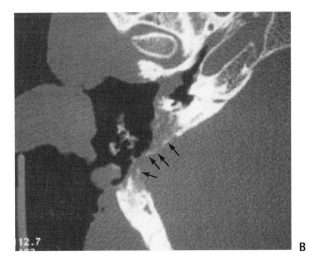

B

Figure 11–1 Computed tomography (CT) of squamous cell carcinoma (SCCA) of the external auditory canal **(A,B)**. Axial CT reconstructed in bone algorithm shows an aggressive soft tissue mass (M) destroying the external auditory canal and mastoid air cells. The mass extends anteriorly to involve the squamous portion of the temporal bone (*large arrow*). The mass extends posteriorly into the mastoid bone, and there is early erosion of the bony covering of the transverse sinus (*small arrows*).

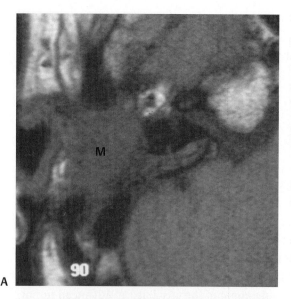

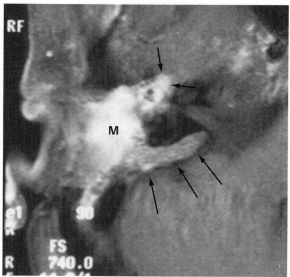

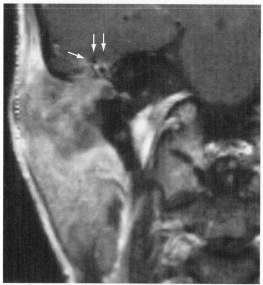

Figure 11–2 Magnetic resonance (MR) of SCCA of the external auditory canal. Axial precontrast **(A)** and postcontrast **(B)** enhanced T1-weighted image of the skull base shows an aggressively intermediate-signal mass (M) that markedly enhances. The lesion invades the middle ear cavity and abuts the middle cranial fossa (*intermediate-length arrows*). The tumor abuts the vestibule (*small arrow*) and is in close proximity to the cochlea. This aggressive tumor extends into the medial portion of the petrous apex (*long arrows*). **(C)** Coronal contrast-enhanced CT in a different patient shows the tumor extending through the tegmen and into the middle cranial fossa (*arrows*).

images can demonstrate asymmetric thickening and enhancement of the facial nerve in its mastoid or tympanic segment, indicating its involvement. If potential involvement of the facial nerve is suspected, careful examination of its entire course should be performed to look for retrograde as well as antegrade perineural spread.

If the vascular structures (i.e., internal carotid artery and the jugular vein) appear to be involved on MRI or CT, further assessment with MRI angiography and MRI venography or sometimes conventional angiography may be indicated. On MRI angiographic studies, vascular involvement is seen as vessel wall irregularity, vessel narrowing, or the presence of filling defects (**Fig. 11–2**).

Angiography

If the internal carotid artery is suspected to be involved by EAC carcinoma, angiography with ipsilateral balloon occlusion may be needed to demonstrate the adequacy of cerebral blood flow from the contralateral carotid artery. If the patient is able to tolerate the test occlusion of the carotid artery, it may be sacrificed by endovascular procedure or at the time of the surgery. On the other hand, failed test occlusion may necessitate performance of extracranial to intracranial bypass before the surgical resection of the tumor. During angiography, it is important to pay careful attention to the venous outflow phase to determine the adequacy of the contralateral sigmoid/jugular system in case the surgery requires sacrifice of the sigmoid sinus or internal jugular vein.

PEARLS _____

- In early-stage squamous cell carcinomas of EAC, nonspecific soft tissue thickening or polypoid mass is seen on CT and MRI.
- Extension to the bone with erosion and gross bone destruction is best detected by high-resolution bone algorithm CT.
- Local extension into the parotid space, temporomandibular (TM) joint, middle ear, and mastoid cavity may be detected on CT or MRI. Invasion of otic capsule (inner ear) is very uncommon.
- Facial nerve involvement can be assessed with CT or MRI, although MRI is more sensitive in detecting nerve involvement and perineural spread.
- If the involvement of carotid artery or jugular vein is suspected, additional evaluation with magnetic resonance angiography/venography (MRA/MRV) or conventional angiography with test balloon occlusion of carotid artery is needed for surgical planning.

Suggested Readings

Arriaga M. Staging proposal for external auditory meatus carcinoma based on preoperative clinical examination and computed tomography findings. Ann Otol Rhinol Laryngol 1990;99:714–721

Arriaga M, Curtin HD, Takahashi H, Kamerer DB. The role of preoperative CT scans in staging external auditory meatus carcinoma: radiologic-pathologic correlation study. Otolaryngol Head Neck Surg 1991;105:6–11

Arriaga M, Hirsch BE, Kamerer DB. Squamous cell carcinoma of the external auditory meatus (canal). Otolaryngol Head Neck Surg 1989;101:330–337

Goodwin WJ, Jesse RH. Malignant neoplasms of the external auditory canal. Arch Otolaryngol 1980;106:675–679

Hirsch BE, Myers EN, Moody SA. Malignant tumors of the temporal bone. In: Laercio O, Selaimen S, eds. Otologia Clinia e Cirurgica. Revinter: Tijuca, Brazil 2000:319–329

Maya MM, Lo WWM, Kovanlikaya I. Temporal bone tumors and cerebellopontine angle lesions. In: Som PM, Curtin HD, eds. Head and Neck Imaging, 4th ed. St. Louis: Mosby, 2003:1275–1374

CHAPTER 12 Basal Cell Carcinoma
Vaishali Phalke

Epidemiology

Carcinomas of the external auditory canal (EAC) are rare. Basal cell carcinoma is not as common as squamous cell carcinoma, which is by far the most common tumor of the ear.

Clinical Features

Basal cell carcinomas in this region most commonly arise in the pinna or postauricular sulcus and extend into the EAC along the skin or along the cartilage. The middle ear cavity is very rarely affected. Bilateral basal cell carcinoma has been reported in Gorlin-Goltz syndrome, which is a cancer predisposition syndrome characterized by multiple basal cell carcinomas and diverse developmental defects. The basal cell carcinoma may present as ulcerated lesions or as tumor masses involving the EAC. It may present with progressive hearing loss, with involvement of cranial nerves V and VII, or it may even be asymptomatic. Metastasis may occur to the parotid gland and lymph nodes.

Pathology

Histologic appearance consists of islands of atypical basal cells, with neoplastic cells resembling normal basal cells with large basophilic oval nuclei, and a peripheral palisade arrangement.

Treatment

Basal cell carcinoma is an aggressive disease and prompt radical surgery is recommended. Early tumors can be treated with Mohs' surgery. Some reports suggest that adjuvant radiation therapy appears to offer better local control. Unlike squamous cell carcinoma, it is very unusual for basal call carcinoma to metastasize to the primary-echelon draining lymph nodes. As a result, resection of the local disease is

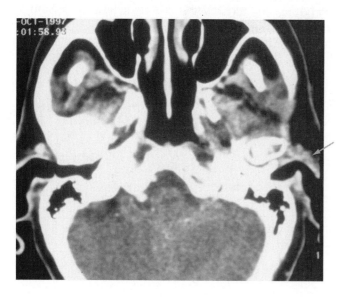

Figure 12–1 Axial contrast computed tomography (CT) shows early basal cell carcinoma infiltrating the tragus and pretragal region (*arrow*). Compare this involvement to the normal appearance of this region on the uninvolved side.

usually adequate. However, basal cell carcinomas may be intermixed with squamous cell carcinomas. These "mixed" lesions may metastasize to the lymph nodes and require treatment of the appropriate nodal groups.

Imaging Findings

CT

If locally invasive, there may be bony involvement of the external auditory canal or temporomandibular joint, which may be seen in the form of infiltrative erosive changes within the involved bones. Lytic destruction of the middle ear, mastoid, and petrous part of the temporal bone in advanced case has been reported (**Fig. 12–1** and **Fig. 12–2**).

MRI

These lesions are intermediate signal on T1 and T2 and homogeneously enhance with contrast. Advanced lesions may extend to the underlying bone.

PEARLS _____

- The imaging findings are nonspecific and the role of imaging is to evaluate the local spread of tumor.
- Perineural spread is very rare in pure basal call carcinomas, but may be seen in lesions in which basal cell carcinoma is associated with squamous cell carcinomas

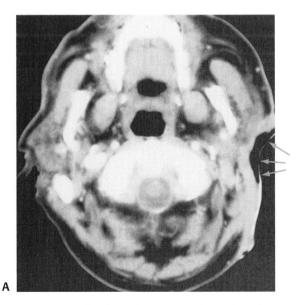 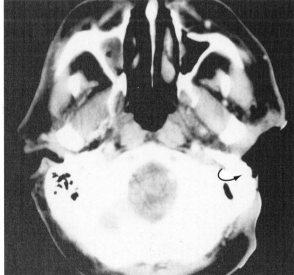

A   B

Figure 12–2 (A,B) Axial contrast-enhanced studies performed through the region of the external auditory canal show a more advanced and ulcerated basal cell carcinoma arising from the periauricular region (*straight arrows*). The mass extends deeply to the cortex of the mastoid bone (*curved arrow*).

Suggested Readings

Lobo CJ, Timms MS, Puranik VC. Basal cell carcinoma of the external auditory canal and Gorlin-Goltz syndrome: a case report. J Laryngol Otol 1997;111:850–851

Mann SB, Yande R, Arora MM, Dutta BN. Bilateral basal cell carcinoma of the ears. (A case report). J Laryngol Otol 1982;96:951–954

Vandeweyer E, Thill MP, Deraemaecker R. Basal cell carcinoma of the external auditory canal. Acta Chir Belg 2002;102:137–140

CHAPTER 13 Melanoma
Vaishali Phalke

Epidemiology

Primary melanoma may occur on any skin surface where melanocytes normally or abnormally are present. Melanoma of the pinna compromises 7 to 14% of all melanomas of the head and neck, though it is extremely rare to have involvement of the external auditory canal. Involvement of the cutaneous surfaces most commonly occurs on the helix or the antihelix of the pinna or in the region of the external auditory meatus, as these regions receive intense sun exposure. The mean age at diagnosis for head and neck melanomas tends to between 60 and 70 years of age. Tumors involving ears are more common in males than females.

Clinical Features

Involvement of the external auditory meatus may either represent extensive lesions that originate in the pinna and extend into the external auditory canal, or primarily involve the meatus of the external auditory canal. Primary involvement of the canal has only rarely been reported. Most cases present with hearing loss and otorrhea. The lesion on physical examination may represent a dark fleshy mass or a pink-gray polypoidal mass.

Pathology

Staging of melanomas is based on the tumor, node, metastasis (TNM) classification. The primary tumor (T) is subdivided as follows: Tx, primary tumor cannot be assessed; T0, no evidence of primary tumor; Tis, melanoma in situ; T1, melanoma is 1.0 mm in thickness; T2, melanoma is 1.01 to 2.0 mm; T3, melanoma is 2.01 to 4.0 mm; and T4, melanoma is >4.0 mm.

As defined by Wallace Clark, the level of invasion with regard to the papillary dermis, reticular dermis, and subcutis is used to define subcategories of T1 melanomas, but it is not used not for thicker melanomas. Poor outcome is predicted by increasing thickness of the lesion. Histologic examination identifies sheets and nests of atypical melanocytes. The cells can have large pleomorphic nuclei with prominent nucleoli. The cytoplasm can have considerable amounts of melanin pigment. Prognosis is worst for lesions of the external auditory canal due to a delay in diagnosis and a greater propensity for metastatic disease. Tumors in the external auditory meatus drain primarily to the intraparotid and upper cervical (level II) and posterior cervical (level V) lymph node groups.

Treatment

Treatment entails wide local incision and lateral temporal bone resection alone or in combination with radiation therapy. It has also been combined with various dissections of the neck lymph nodes and parotid nodal dissection to treat primary-echelon nodal drainage sites.

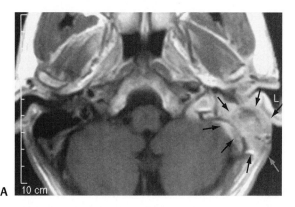
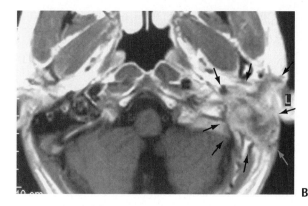

Figure 13–1 **(A)** Contrast-enhanced T1-weighted image shows an aggressive enhancing mass involving the posterior peri-auricular region (*arrows*). **(B)** The tumor extends inferiorly to invade the parotid gland (*arrows*).

Imaging Findings

CT

Computed tomography demonstrates a soft tissue mass involving the pinna, which may extend into the external auditory canal. Aggressive tumors may erode the cortical bone of the external auditory canal.

MRI

These lesions are intermediate signal on T1 and T2 and diffusely enhance with contrast. Advanced lesions may extend superiorly along the scalp and extend inferiorly into the pretragal region and involve the superior portion of the parotid gland (**Fig. 13–1**).

PEARLS

- The imaging findings are nonspecific.
- Imaging is used to search for occult bony destruction of the underlying calvarium or external auditory canal.
- Perineural spread is unusual in melanoma but may be seen in the desmoplastic subtype.

Suggested Readings

Balch CM, Soong SJ, Atkins MB, et al. An evidence-based staging system for cutaneous melanoma. CA Cancer J Clin 2004;54:131–149

Gillgren P, Månsson-Brahme E, Frisell J, et al. Epidemiological characteristics of cutaneous malignant melanoma of the head and neck. Acta Oncol 1999;38:1069–1074

Kang S, Barnhill RL, Graeme-Cook F, Randolph G, Nadol JB, Sober AJ. Primary malignant melanoma of the external auditory canal: a case report with presentation as an aural polyp. Am J Otol 1992;13:194–196

Langman A, Yarington T, Patterson SD. Malignant melanoma of the external auditory canal. Otolaryngol Head Neck Surg 1996;114:645–648

Milbrath MM, Campbell BH, Madiedo G, Janjan NA. Malignant melanoma of the external auditory canal. Am J Clin Oncol 1998;21:28–30

CHAPTER 14 Ossicular Malformations

Ashok Srinivasan

Epidemiology

Ossicular malformations are commonly associated with external auditory canal (EAC) malformations due to similar embryologic origins (for the auricle, first and second branchial arches; for the EAC, first branchial cleft; for the ossicular chain except stapes footplate, first and second branchial arches). Isolated ossicular malformations without outer ear abnormalities are rare but occur. Although autosomal dominant inheritance has been reported in some cases, these anomalies can be seen in association with such syndromes as Goldenhar and Treacher Collins.

Clinical Features

The outer ear anomalies that can be seen include microtia and atresia or stenosis of the EAC. In the presence of EAC abnormalities, there is an increased incidence of primary and secondary cholesteatomas. The ossicular malformations primarily produce a conductive type of hearing loss due to loss of sound transmission.

Pathology

Ossicular malformations have variable appearances on pathology that include hypoplasia, aplasia, or shortening of either a part of an ossicle or the entire ossicle itself. There can also be abnormal union between ossicles.

Treatment

Congenital conductive hearing loss due to ossicular deformities can be treated by either rehabilitation with a hearing aid or surgical reconstruction using a variety of ossicular prostheses.

Imaging Findings

CT

The ossicles most commonly malformed or absent include the stapes and incus. The stapes can reveal aplasia, hypoplasia, absence of head and crura, fusion of head to promontory, fixation of the footplate, and a columnar type deformity. Anomalies of the incus include aplasia, shortening, or malformation of the long process, absent or fibrous union of the incudostapedial joint, and fusion of the short process to the lateral semicircular canal. The malleus can be aplastic or have a deformed head. There can also be fusion at the incudomalleal joint or manubrium of the malleus, with the long process of the incus and the head of the stapes. Congenital fixation of the malleal head to the lateral epitympanic wall, called the malleus bar, is a rare anomaly.

The facial nerve anomalies associated with ossicular malformations are displacement and bony dehiscence of the tympanic segment. The nerve can be displaced inferiorly and medially and often crosses the oval window. Congenital absence of the oval window has been reported with these facial

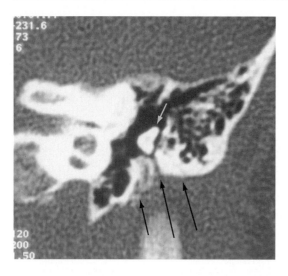

Figure 14–1 Coronal computed tomography (CT) through the temporal bone shows bony external auditory canal (EAC) atresia (*arrows*). There is incomplete separation of the incudomalleolar joint with resultant fusion of the anlage (*small arrow*). The anlage is also laterally displaced. EAC atresia is commonly associated with ossicular malformations of the malleus and incus due to their common embryologic precursors.

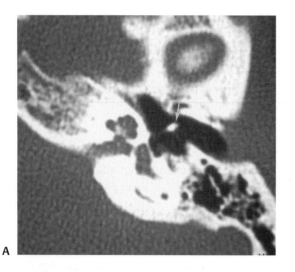

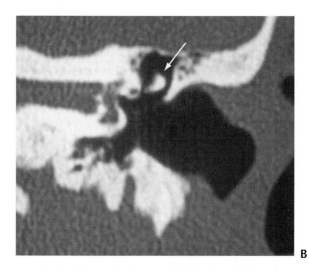

FFigure 14–2 (A) Axial and **(B)** coronal images through the temporal bone performed in a patient with conductive hearing loss show isolated absence of the incus and the stapes.

The *arrow* points to the malleus. However, the incus and the stapes are not seen.

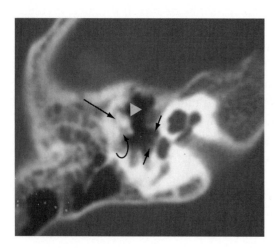

Figure 14–3 Axial CT obtained in a patient with Goldenhar syndrome with an EAC atresia that shows lateralization of the malleus and incus. The head of the malleus and short process of the incus directly abut and are partially fused with the lateral wall of the epitympanum (*long arrow*). In addition, there appears to be incomplete development of the incudomalleolar joint with resultant partial fusion of the head of the malleus (*arrowhead*) and short process of the incus (*curved arrow*). The anterior and posterior crura of the stapes are visualized (*short arrows*).

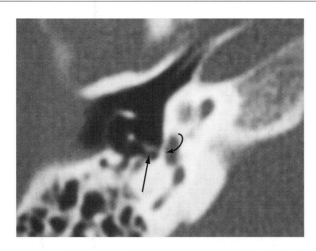

Figure 14–4 Monopod stapes. Axial CT through the oval window demonstrates only one crux of the stapes to be present. The posterior crux is present (*straight arrow*) but the anterior crux is absent. This is characteristic of a monopod stapes. In addition, there appears to be a complete bony covering of the oval window (*curved arrow*), suggesting aplasia of the oval window.

nerve anomalies, presumably from a mechanical barrier to contact of the stapes footplate with the otic capsule, which induces oval window formation (**Fig. 14–1, Fig. 14–2, Fig. 14–3,** and **Fig. 14–4**).

MRI

Magnetic resonance is of no additional benefit in the diagnosis and characterization of ossicular malformations. It can be useful for assessing any associated inner ear anomalies.

PEARLS _____

- Ossicular malformations are commonly associated with external ear anomalies.
- There is an increased incidence of cholesteatoma in the presence of external ear abnormalities.

Suggested Readings

Jahrsdoerfer RA. Embryology of the facial nerve. Am J Otol 1988;9:423–426

Jahrsdoerfer RA. The facial nerve in congenital middle ear malformations. Laryngoscope 1981;91:1217–1225

Kurosaki Y, Tanaka YO, Itai Y. Malleus bar as a rare cause of congenital malleus fixation: CT demonstration. AJNR Am J Neuroradiol 1998;19:1229–1230

Sando I, Shibahara Y, Takagi A, Takahara T, Yamaguchi N. Frequency and localization of congenital anomalies of the middle and inner ears: a human temporal bone histopathological study. Int J Pediatr Otorhinolaryngol 1988;16:1–22

Staecker H, Merchant SN. Temporal bone pathology case of the month. Congenital fixation of the incus. Am J Otol 2000;21:137–138

Subotic R, Mladina R, Risavi R. Congenital bony fixation of the malleus. Acta Otolaryngol 1998;118:833–836

Yokoyama T, Iino Y, Kakizaki K, Murakami Y. Human temporal bone study on the postnatal ossification process of auditory ossicles. Laryngoscope 1999;109:927–930

Zeifer B, Sabini P, Sonne J. Congenital absence of the oval window: radiologic diagnosis and associated anomalies. AJNR Am J Neuroradiol 2000;21:322–327

CHAPTER 15 Congenital Cholesteatoma

Sachin Gujar

Etiology

Congenital cholesteatomas are distinct from acquired cholesteatomas of the middle ear. Previously thought to be rare, they are being more frequently diagnosed in young children. Congenital cholesteatomas are known to develop in four temporal bone sites: the petrous apex, the middle ear, the mastoid, and the external auditory canal. Some can affect both the middle ear and the mastoid. We limit our discussion here to middle ear lesions, as other locations are discussed elsewhere in this book.

The current established criteria for diagnosis for a congenital cholesteatoma was described in 1986 by Levenson et al, who modified the original criteria of Derlacki and Clemis from 1965. The criteria now include a sac medial to an intact tympanic membrane in a patient who has never had a previous tympanic membrane perforation, otorrhea, or prior otologic surgery. Prior otitis media does not completely exclude the diagnosis. These lesions are most often unilateral, though bilateral lesions have been reported.

Several mechanisms have been proposed to explain the pathogenesis of congenital cholesteatoma, including persistent epidermoid cell rest, ingrowth of meatal epidermis, and reflux of amniotic fluid. Of these, the favored theory of pathogenesis appears to be the persistence and continued growth of the epidermoid formation that normally exists in the middle ear during fetal life and usually disappears after 33 weeks of gestation. The theory also explains the more common anterior-superior quadrant location of these lesions.

Clinical Features

Congenital cholesteatomas are often asymptomatic, and detected incidentally at routine pediatric otologic examination. On otologic exam, they appear as a white mass behind an intact tympanic membrane, a feature that helps differentiate them from acquired cholesteatomas. However, they may result in conductive hearing loss, if they are large or in contact with the ossicular chain.

Pathology

The gross appearance of a congenital cholesteatoma may take one of two forms: (1) the closed keratinous cyst; and (2) the open form of the lesion, with multiple layers of keratinous squames carpeted by cholesteatoma matrix that covers a part of the middle ear surface. Microscopically, the lesion resembles other epidermoid inclusion cysts with stratified squamous epithelium, exfoliated keratinized material, and a cholesterol-rich content.

Treatment

Congenital cholesteatomas are treated surgically. Early surgery and long follow-up are suggested.

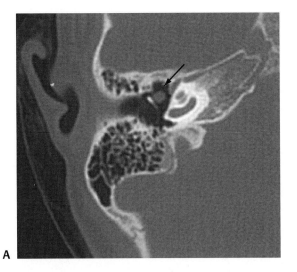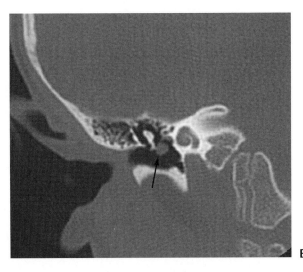

A   B

Figure 15–1 (A,B) Axial and coronal images of a thin-section temporal bone computed tomography (CT) show a well-defined soft tissue nodule (*arrows*) medial to the ossicular plane consistent with a congenital cholesteatoma.

Imaging Findings

CT

A small middle ear cholesteatoma presents as a well-circumscribed nodular mass, most often in the superior anterior quadrant of the middle ear. The other common locations are the posterior epitympanum and peristapedial regions. Larger lesions may be associated with bone and ossicular erosions, though less commonly as compared with acquired cholesteatoma. Ossicular erosion is uncommon with anterior mesotympanic lesions, but facial nerve canal erosion may occur. Posterior lesions are often associated with more extensive disease, with conductive hearing loss due to their proximity to the ossicular chain, and with recidivism. Involvement of the aditus ad antrum could result in mastoid opacification (**Fig. 15–1**).

MRI

All cholesteatomas have a nonspecific low to intermediate T1 signal, and intermediate to bright T2 signal. There may be peripheral enhancement around the nonenhancing cholesteatoma due to associated inflammation. Magnetic resonance imaging (MRI) can help in the exclusion of other mass lesions in the differential diagnosis, such as facial schwannoma and glomus tumor, which show enhancement following contrast administration.

PEARLS _____

- Thin-section temporal bone CT is the mainstay of diagnosis. Contrast-enhanced T1 MRI may be complementary if lesions such as glomus tympanicum are in the differential diagnosis.
- Classic congenital cholesteatomas arise medial to the plane formed by the manubrium of the malleus and the long process of the incus, whereas acquired cholesteatoma classically arise in the Prussak space, which is lateral to the ossicular plane.
- CT is also useful in the evaluation of the more extensive lesions, in involvement of the mastoid, and in ossicular and bone erosion.

Suggested Readings

Hudgins PA. Congenital cholesteatoma, middle ear. In: Harnsberger HR, ed. Diagnostic Imaging: Head and Neck. Salt Lake City: Amirsys, 2004:I-2–30

Levenson MJ, Parisier SC, Chute P, Wenig S, Juarbe C. A review of twenty congenital cholesteatomas of the middle ear in children. Otolaryngol Head Neck Surg 1986;94:560–567

Michaels L. An epidermoid formation in the developing middle ear; possible source of cholesteatoma. J Otolaryngol 1986;15:169–174

Swartz JD, Harnsberger HR. The middle ear and mastoid. In: Swartz JD, Harnsberger HR, eds. Imaging of the Temporal Bone, 3rd ed. New York: Thieme, 1998:47–169

CHAPTER 16 Aberrant (Intratympanic) Internal Carotid Artery
Sachin Gujar

Epidemiology

The incidence of an aberrant course of the internal carotid artery (ICA) is less than 1%. More than 60 to 90% of the cases described in the literature occur in females, with a majority occurring on the right side. No explanation for this preponderance is provided in the literature.

Clinical Features

This is an unusual but important condition that may be detected incidentally or may present with pulsatile tinnitus or conductive hearing loss. The aberrant ICA appears as a vascular-appearing bluish retrotympanic mass that resembles a middle ear paraganglioma clinically. This is rarely seen bilaterally. It is important that the diagnosis be made to prevent the disastrous outcome of an inadvertent biopsy or surgical injury.

Pathology

Embryologically, an aberrant ICA appears to occur when there is regression or atresia/agenesis of the cervical segment of the ICA, and it is replaced by an enlarged inferior tympanic branch of the ascending pharyngeal artery, which anastomoses with an enlarged caroticotympanic artery. This usually tiny vessel enters the tympanic cavity through the inferior tympanic calculus along with the Jacobson tympanic branch of cranial nerve IX. There is then reconstitution of the petrous ICA via the communication through a dehiscence in the carotid canal.

Treatment

There is no treatment for an aberrant ICA, because it is a rare developmental anomaly that provides a critical anastomosis for intracranial blood flow. As stated above, clinical findings can mimic a glomus tympanicum. Correct diagnosis is important to prevent the disastrous outcome of a biopsy or potentially the endaural resection of a presumed small glomus tumor.

For cases of an aberrant ICA associated with pulsatile tinnitus or hemorrhage, treatment has included interposition of synthetic material or sacrifice of the vessel.

Imaging Findings

CT

The computed tomography (CT) appearance of the aberrant ICA is characteristic. The aberrant ICA is seen to enter the tympanic cavity through an enlarged inferior tympanic canaliculus, which has a more lateral and posterior location than the usual location of vertical segment of the ICA. The aberrant vessel then courses anteriorly across the cochlear promontory to join the horizontal petrous carotid canal through a dehiscence in the carotid canal. On coronal images, this may have the appearance of a focal mass in the hypotympanum, and following this structure on consecutive images will demonstrate the

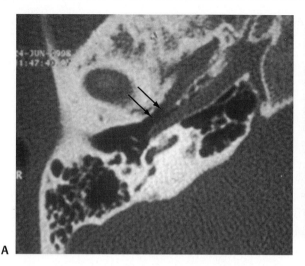

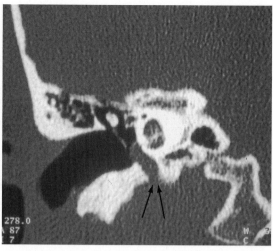

Figure 16–1 Aberrant carotid artery: computed tomography (CT). **(A)** Axial CT through the temporal bone demonstrates the aberrant course of the internal carotid artery. The bony covering of the carotid canal is dehiscent. The carotid artery (*arrows*) extends into the middle ear cavity.

(B) Coronal image obtained in the same patient as in **A** shows the carotid artery to course superiorly through an enlarged inferior tympanic canaliculus (*arrows*) and extend into the middle ear cavity.

tubular nature of the abnormality. Rarely, a persistent stapedial artery may accompany an aberrant internal carotid artery (**Fig. 16–1**).

MRI

The routine pulse sequences are not very helpful in making the diagnosis. However, magnetic resonance angiography (MRA) can be used to make the diagnosis of an aberrant ICA. The source and the projection images from MRA demonstrate the unusual posterolateral course of the ICA at the skull base (**Fig. 16–2**).

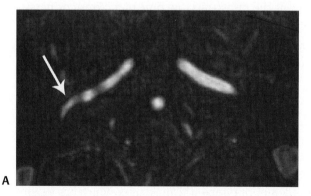

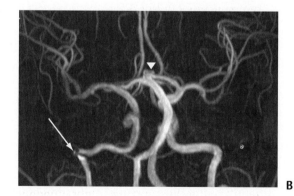

Figure 16–2 Aberrant carotid artery: magnetic resonance angiography (MRA). Axial image from an MRA shows the anomalous course of the internal carotid artery (ICA) (*arrow*). Compare this to the similar appearance of the CT correlate demonstrated in **Fig. 16–1A.** Frontal projection from a maxi-

mum intensity projection MRI angiogram demonstrates the abnormal course and pinched contour of the ICA (*arrow*). Note the incidental anterior communicating artery aneurysm (*arrowhead*).

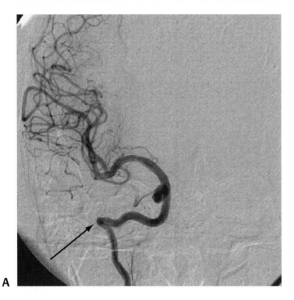

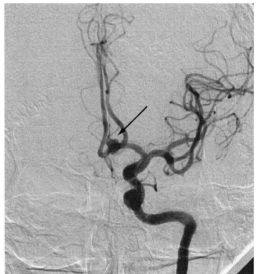

A

B

Figure 16–3 Aberrant carotid artery: conventional angiography. **(A)** Frontal projection of an internal carotid angiogram performed in the same patient illustrated in **Fig. 16–2** shows the characteristic kinked appearance (*arrow*) of the right aberrant ICA. **(B)** Compare this to the normal course of the internal carotid artery on the contralateral side. Again noted is the incidental anterior communicating artery aneurysm (*arrow*).

Angiography

The posterolateral location and the pinched contour of the aberrant vessel results in a characteristic angiographic appearance. Angiography, however, is not necessary for the diagnosis (**Fig. 16–3**).

PEARLS _____

- Clinical distinction from a vascular mass such as glomus tympanicum is often impossible. This is a diagnosis that can be made only on imaging.
- Thin-section temporal bone CT is diagnostic and shows the abnormal lateral location of the carotid canal, with a smaller caliber vessel that traverses the hypotympanum across the cochlear promontory.
- MRI angiography and conventional angiography demonstrate the abnormal posterolateral course of the ICA, with a pinched contour.

Suggested Readings

Davidson HC. Imaging of the temporal bone. Neuroimaging Clin North Am 2004;14:721–760

Harnsberger HR. The temporal bone. In: Harnsberger HR, ed. Handbook of Head and Neck Imaging, 2nd ed. St. Louis: Mosby, 1995:441

Lo WW, Solti-Bowman LG, McElveen JT Jr. Aberrant carotid artery: radiologic diagnosis with emphasis in high-resolution computed tomography. Radiographics 1985;5:985–993

Swartz JD, Harnsberger HR. Temporal bone vascular anatomy, anomalies, and diseases, emphasizing the clinical-radiological problem of pulsatile tinnitus. In: Swartz JD, Harnsberger HR, eds. Imaging of the Temporal Bone, 3rd ed. New York: Thieme, 1997:170

Epidemiology

Persistent stapedial artery (PSA) is a rare congenital vascular anomaly of the middle ear. The prevalence of PSA is 0.02 to 0.05% in surgical series, and it was slightly higher (0.48%) in a temporal bone study.

Clinical Features

The majority of patients are asymptomatic. Rarely, PSA may result in pulsatile tinnitus, conductive hearing loss, or a pulsatile retrotympanic red mass.

Pathology

The stapedial artery arises at 4 to 5 weeks of fetal life from the hyoid artery and connects branches of the future external carotid artery to the internal carotid artery. The hyoid artery is a derivative of the second branchial arch, near its origin from the proximal internal carotid artery (third branchial arch). It extends cranially and passes through the mesenchymal primordium of the stapes (second branchial arch) and forms the obturator foramen of the stapes. The stapedial artery gives rise to two branches after entering the cranial cavity. The upper, or supraorbital, branch becomes the middle meningeal artery and transiently anastomoses with the ophthalmic artery. The lower, or maxillomandibular, division has two branches: mandibular and infraorbital. This lower division leaves the cranial cavity via the foramen spinosum. Normally, anastomoses develop between the ventral pharyngeal arteries (roots of adult external carotid artery) and the lower division branches of the stapedial artery, which involutes during the 10th week of fetal life with reversal of flow at the foramen spinosum level. When the artery fails to involute in the 3rd fetal month, a persistent stapedial artery results. It is usually seen with an aberrant internal carotid artery or other middle ear anomalies, especially of the stapes and facial nerve, and may be bilateral. Other associations with trisomy 13, 15, and 21, otosclerosis, anencephaly, Paget disease, and neurofibromatosis have been reported.

Treatment

This anomaly is often an incidental finding and is left untreated. If a PSA is the presumed cause of tinnitus, surgical ligation or endovascular occlusion may be considered.

Preoperative knowledge of the presence of a PSA is important information for the otologist prior to middle ear exploration or cochlear implant placement.

Imaging Findings

CT

The PSA arises from the petrous part of the internal carotid artery, enters the anteromedial hypotympanum, and is contained in the Jacobson canal. After leaving the osseous canal, it crosses the cochlear promontory and passes through the obturator foramen of the stapes. It then enters the fallopian canal

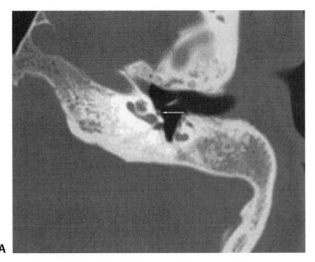
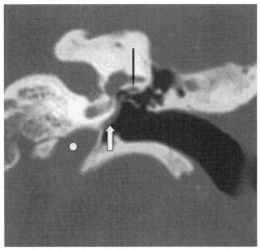

A

B

Figure 17–1 Persistent stapedial artery. **(A)** Axial image of the left temporal bone shows PSA (*white arrow*) coursing over the cochlear promontory. **(B)** Coronal image of left temporal bone shows the origin of the PSA (*white arrow*) from the petrous part of the carotid artery (○) and coursing superiorly along the cochlear promontory. The tympanic portion of the facial nerve (*black arrow*) is also seen.

through a dehiscence just behind the cochleariform process and travels anteriorly in the anterior facial canal. This leads to prominence of the tympanic part of the facial nerve, an indirect imaging sign of PSA. Finally, the PSA exits just before the geniculate ganglion, entering into the extradural space of the middle cranial fossa. Another indirect sign of PSA is absent or hypoplastic foramen spinosum, though the foramen spinosum can be congenitally absent in 3.2% of the population, and hence other imaging signs of PSA need to be present to confirm its presence (**Fig. 17–1**).

MRI

Magnetic resonance imaging is nondiagnostic. Magnetic resonance angiography may show absent middle meningeal artery.

Cerebral Angiography

External carotid angiography shows the absence of a normal middle meningeal artery. Internal carotid angiography shows the presence of a persistent stapedial artery arising from either the intrapetrosal portion of the internal carotid artery or the aberrant internal carotid artery.

PEARLS _____

- High-resolution temporal bone CT is diagnostic.
- One needs to differentiate a PSA from a facial nerve tumor such as hemangioma/schwannoma.
- A reddish pulsatile mass behind the tympanic membrane entails the clinical differential diagnosis of glomus tympanicum tumor, aberrant carotid artery, or PSA.

Suggested Readings

Boscia R, Knox RD, Adkins WY, Holgate RC. Persistent stapedial artery supplying a glomus tympanicum tumor. Arch Otolaryngol Head Neck Surg 1990;116:852–854

Davies DG. Persistent stapedial artery: a temporal bone report. J Laryngol Otol 1967;81:649–660

Ginsberg LE, Pruett SW, Chen MY, et al. Skull base foramina of the middle cranial fossa: reassessment of normal variation with high resolution CT. AJNR Am J Neuroradiol 1994;15:283–291

Govaerts PJ, Marquet TF, Cremers CWRJ, et al. Persistent stapedial artery: does it prevent successful surgery? Ann Otol Rhinol Laryngol 1993;102:724–728

Guinto FC, Garrabrant EC, Radcliffe WB. Radiology of the persistent stapedial artery. Radiology 1972;105:365–369

Roll JD, Urban MA, Larson TC, et al. Bilateral aberrant internal carotid arteries with bilateral persistent stapedial arteries and bilateral duplicated internal carotid arteries. AJNR Am J Neuroradiol 2003;24:762–765

Silbergleit R, Quint DJ, Mehta BA, Patel SC, Metes JJ, Noujaim SE. The persistent stapedial artery. AJNR Am J Neuroradiol 2000;21:572–577

Steffen TN. Vascular anomalies of the middle ear. Laryngoscope 1968;78:171–197

Sachin Gujar

Epidemiology

In the literature, the reported incidence of a dehiscent jugular bulb varies from 2 to 7%.

Clinical Features

Dehiscence of the jugular bulb may be seen as a bluish vascular retrotympanic mass in the posteroinferior quadrant of the tympanic membrane, when viewed with an otoscope. This may present with venous pulsatile tinnitus or as an asymptomatic mass that cannot be differentiated from a paraganglioma clinically. Associated conductive hearing loss secondary to ossicular impingement is rare.

Pathology

A dehiscent jugular bulb is a congenital variant that can present as a vascular pseudomass in the middle ear. Dehiscence is defined by absence of the bony canal wall between the lateral aspect of the jugular foramen and middle ear cavity.

The jugular bulb variations that commonly occur include an asymmetrically large jugular bulb, a high-riding jugular bulb with or without dehiscence, and a jugular diverticulum. An asymmetrically large jugular bulb is a common finding and is not thought to be a cause of symptoms. In the asymmetrically large jugular bulb, the right jugular bulb is larger twice as often as on the left side.

The top of the jugular bulb is defined by the most cephalad extension of the bulb reaching above the floor of the internal auditory canal. At our institution, a high-riding jugular bulb is described if the top of the jugular bulb is above the basal turn of the cochlea.

If a jugular bulb is dehiscent, it can present as a vascular retrotympanic mass commonly seen behind the posteroinferior quadrant of the tympanic membrane. The size of the mass depends on the size of the deficiency in the sigmoid plate of the mastoid. This is best diagnosed on computed tomography (CT). When a finger-like projection of the jugular bulb projects cephalad within the petrous temporal bone, a jugular bulb diverticulum is diagnosed. Pulsatile tinnitus can occur due to turbulence of venous flow with this venous variant.

Treatment

No treatment is required for the asymptomatic jugular bulb dehiscence. Treatment may be required if there is inadvertent injury to the bulb. Defects can be treated by occlusion with bone wax, gelatin sponge, or surgical packing. Some cases may require sacrifice of the vein.

Imaging Findings

CT

Computed tomography shows absence of the bony covering of the jugular foramen between the lateral aspect of the jugular foramen and the middle ear cavity (**Fig. 18–1**).

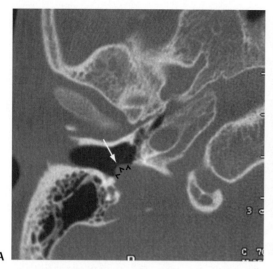
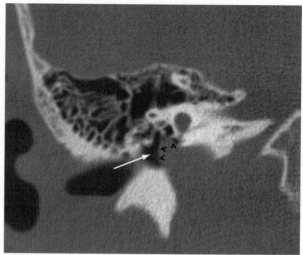

A   B

Figure 18–1 Dehiscent jugular bulb with jugular diverticulum. **(A)** Axial and **(B)** coronal computed tomography (CT) image of the temporal bone shows absence of the medial bony covering (*arrowheads*) of the jugular foramen. Note the focal protrusion of the jugular bulb (*arrow*) extending into the middle ear cavity. This is characteristic of a jugular diverticulum.

MRI

The high-riding jugular bulb can simulate a lesion on contrast-enhanced magnetic resonance imaging (MRI), but MRI venography or CT can be used to confirm the normal venous variant. A bony dehiscence cannot be detected or excluded on MRI, but a lateral lobulation of the jugular bulb on the coronal MRI images may suggest the presence of a dehiscence.

PEARLS

- A high-riding jugular bulb is diagnosed when the top of the jugular foramen is seen at the level of the basal turn of the cochlea. In general, this rule works well; however, this relationship can be variable and may be dependent on the scan angle.
- CT demonstrates the osseous defect over the dehiscent jugular bulb. Contrast-enhanced CT or MRI demonstrates the bulging venous lumen into the middle ear cavity.

Suggested Readings

Harnsberger HR. The temporal bone. In: Harnsberger HR, ed. Handbook of Head and Neck Imaging, 2nd ed. St. Louis: Mosby, 1995:441

Swartz JD, Harnsberger HR. Temporal bone vascular anatomy, anomalies, and diseases, emphasizing the clinical-radiological problem of pulsatile tinnitus. In: Swartz JD, Harnsberger HR, eds. Imaging of the Temporal Bone, 3rd ed. New York: Thieme, 1997:170

19 Acute Otitis Media and Mastoiditis

Ellen G. Hoeffner

Epidemiology

Acute otitis media (AOM) and mastoiditis are infectious processes of the middle ear and a variable portion of the mastoid air cell system. They primarily affect infants and young children. AOM is often preceded by a viral upper respiratory infection that disrupts the mucosal barrier of the nose and nasopharynx, allowing bacteria to adhere and grow. Reflux of infected secretions from the nasopharynx to the eustachian tube allows bacteria to gain entrance to the middle ear.

Clinical Features

Varying degrees of otalgia are usually present, along with fever, sleeplessness, and irritability. Early in the disease process, otoscopy reveals erythema and edema of the tympanic membrane. Fluid rapidly develops in the middle ear, with fluid progressing from serous to purulent. Bulging of the tympanic membrane then occurs with loss of normal bone landmarks. The tympanic membrane may rupture, resulting in decompression of the middle ear and otorrhea. Mastoid tenderness is a common feature. Variable conductive hearing loss may be present.

Pathology

The most common pathogens are *Streptococcus pneumoniae, Haemophilus influenzae,* and *Moraxella catarrhalis.* Strains of bacteria resistant to antibiotics have emerged, especially resistant strains of *S. pneumoniae.*

Pathologic findings consist of mucosal inflammation of the eustachian tube, middle ear, and tympanic membrane. Polymorphonuclear and lymphocytic infiltrates are present along with a mucositis and periostitis. Swelling and thickening of the tympanic membrane occurs and may spread to involve the ear canal. Bone involvement develops if treatment is inadequate.

Treatment

Antibiotics alone are curative in most patients. In uncomplicated cases, myringotomy may be helpful in alleviating pain and quickening resolution of the disease process, whereas it is a critical therapeutic step in the management of complicated cases.

Imaging Findings

CT

Opacification of the middle ear cavity and mastoid air cells with fluid and nonspecific debris is seen in acute uncomplicated otitis and mastoiditis. The integrity of osseous structures, including the ossicles, mastoid cortical bone, and mastoid trabeculae, is preserved.

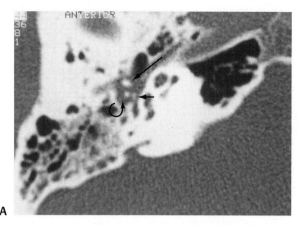
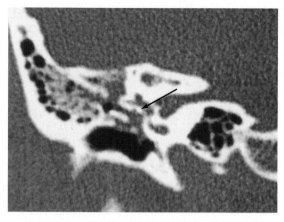

A

B

Figure 19–1 Acute otitis media associated with facial nerve palsy. **(A)** Axial computed tomography (CT) demonstrates mucosal thickening involving the middle ear cavity. The visualized portions of the manubrium of the malleus (*long straight arrow*), the long process of the incus (*curved arrow*), and the stapes (*short straight arrow*) are intact. The imaging findings are nonspecific, and the diagnosis of acute otitis media is based on clinical examination. **(B)** Coronal images show mucosal thickening of the middle ear cavity. The inflammatory process surrounds the tympanic segment (*arrow*) of the facial nerve, resulting in the facial nerve palsy.

Spread of infection to the bone with erosion of the mastoid septa, lateral mastoid cortex, or cortex over the sigmoid plate is termed coalescent mastoiditis. High-resolution computed tomography (CT) is the optimal imaging modality to search for evidence of bone erosion.

Subperiosteal abscess can develop, particularly if there is destruction of the external mastoid cortex. Such abscesses may be postauricular, spread toward the external auditory canal or along the zygomatic bone. Erosion at the mastoid tip may allow infection to spread into the neck, deep to the fascial planes surrounding the sternocleidomastoid and trapezius muscles, with formation of what has been termed a Bezold abscess. This is a life-threatening condition, because the abscess can spread to the larynx and mediastinum and surgical drainage is indicated.

Petrous apicitis results from spread of the infection anteriorly in the temporal bone into a pneumatized petrous apex. Clinically such patients may present with the triad of otorrhea, sixth nerve palsy due to involvement at the level of the Dorello canal, and facial pain secondary to gasserian ganglion irritation. This triad, which is variably present, is referred to as Gradenigo syndrome. Erosive changes of the petrous apex are present on CT (**Fig. 19–1**).

MRI

Acute otitis and mastoiditis are visualized on magnetic resonance imaging (MRI) as nonspecific middle ear and mastoid fluid. The osseous temporal bone structures are poorly visualized on MRI, and this modality should not be used to assess for bone changes such as erosion or destruction. Subperiosteal and Bezold abscesses can be visualized with MRI as a rim enhancing fluid collection.

Magnetic resonance imaging is more useful at searching for intracranial complications than for bone destruction. Epidural, subdural, and intracerebral abscesses can develop via direct extension, hematogenous spread, or thrombophlebitis. Epidural abscess usually occurs in the posterior fossa, with the middle cranial fossa being less common; whereas subdural abscesses or empyemas usually develop along the interhemispheric fissure or tentorium cerebelli. The temporal lobe and cerebellum are the most common locations for intracerebral abscesses developing secondary to otomastoiditis. Meningitis may also develop as a complication that can be seen as leptomeningeal enhancement on MRI.

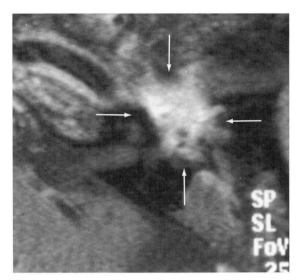

Figure 19–2 Acute otitis media. Axial fat-suppressed contrast-enhanced T1-weighted image shows diffuse enhancement of the middle ear phlegmon (*arrows*) in a patient with advanced acute otitis media. Middle ear fluid associated with less severe serous otitis media does not typically enhance.

Inflammatory debris in contact with the sigmoid sinus may result in thrombophlebitis and dural sinus thrombosis. In over half of such cases, an epidural abscess precedes the development of dural sinus thrombosis. Enhanced CT or MRI may demonstrate the thrombus as a filling defect in the sinus, whereas noncontrast MRI may reveal loss of normal flow void in the sinus on spin-echo images and absence of flow-related enhancement on gradient-echo images. MRI venography, including phase-contrast, time-of-flight, and postcontrast techniques, can demonstrate the thrombus in the vessel, as can newer CT venography techniques. Thrombus can propagate into the transverse and superior sagittal sinuses, the internal jugular vein, and the superior petrosal and cavernous sinuses. Venous infarcts may result from dural sinus thrombosis.

Labyrinthitis may also be a complication of acute otomastoiditis, with infection spreading via the oval or round windows or through direct invasion of the bony labyrinth. Contrast enhancement within the membranous labyrinth can be seen on postcontrast T1-weighted images. Advanced disease may also affect the facial nerve resulting in facial nerve palsy. This may result in abnormal enhancement of the nerve following gadolinium administration (**Fig. 19–2**).

PEARLS _____

- In uncomplicated cases of acute otomastoiditis, nonspecific middle ear and mastoid opacification is seen on CT and MRI.
- Extension to the bone with erosion and resultant coalescent mastoiditis or petrous apicitis is best detected by CT.
- Subperiosteal or Bezold abscesses can be diagnosed with CT or MRI.
- Many intracranial complications can be diagnosed with either CT or MRI, although MRI is generally thought to be more useful for intracranial pathology, particularly subtle findings such as meningitis.
- Diagnosis of dural sinus thrombosis may require MRI or CT venography, whereas labyrinthitis can be diagnosed on postcontrast T1-weighted images.

Suggested Readings

Antonelli PJ, Garside JA, Mancuso AA, et al. Computed tomography and the diagnosis of coalescent mastoiditis. Otolaryngol Head Neck Surg 1999;120:350–354

Canalis RF, Lambert PR. Acute suppurative otitis media and mastoiditis. In: Canalis RF, Lambert PR, eds. The Ear: Comprehensive Otology. Philadelphia: Lippincott Williams & Wilkins, 2000:397–408

Maroldi R, Farina D, Palvarini A, et al. Computed tomography and magnetic resonance imaging of pathologic conditions of the middle ear. Eur J Radiol 2001;40:78–93

Migirov L. Computed tomographic verses surgical findings in complicated acute otomastoiditis. Ann Otol Rhinol Laryngol 2003;112:675–677

Nemzek WR, Swartz JD. Temporal bone: inflammatory disease. In: Som PM, Curtin HD, eds. Head and Neck Imaging, 4th ed. St. Louis: Mosby, 2003:1173–1229

Vazquez E, Castellote A, Piqueras J, et al. Imaging of complications of acute mastoiditis in children. Radiographics 2003;23:359–372

CHAPTER 20 Chronic Otitis Media

Ellen G. Hoeffner

Epidemiology

Chronic otitis media (COM) is an unresolved inflammatory process of the middle ear and mastoid. Early theories proposed that eustachian tube dysfunction was the primary cause of COM. Such dysfunction was thought to lead to collapse of the eustachian tube and result in negative intratympanic pressure. This resulted in fluid transudation and accumulation of fluid in the middle ear cavity. More recent data suggests that there is also likely an infectious etiology, as COM generally begins as an acute middle ear infection that can persist and evolve over time.

Clinical Features

Clinically, patients complain of otorrhea and hearing loss. Hearing loss is usually conductive, although a sensorineural component may be present in advanced cases. Patients with COM may have middle ear mucosal proliferation, which predisposes the formation of acquired cholesteatoma. Effusions may be serous, mucoid, or purulent. Patients may also complain of otalgia during acute exacerbations. On otoscopic examination, the eardrum may be retracted or perforated. There may also be tympanosclerosis. Associated abnormalities include cholesteatoma (with or without ossicular erosion), granulomas, or polyps.

Pathology

While the effusions associated with COM may be of variable consistency, bacteria are usually present. *Pseudomonas aeruginosa* is the most common bacteria, being present in 40 to 65% of cases, with *Staphylococcus aureus* present in 10 to 20%. Anaerobic bacteria are also frequent pathogens in COM, being found in 8 to 59% of patients. Over half the cases of COM may be polymicrobial.

These pathogens, along with the chronic effusion, induce changes in the middle ear mucosa, including a chronic inflammation and granulation tissue. Middle ear mucosal hyperplasia and formation of gland-like structures in the submucosa can occur, with the latter being responsible for the persistent effusions. These changes can be extensive and irreversible. Adhesions and scars can form in quiescent periods. Ossicular erosions may result from direct infection, vascular thrombosis, and subsequent necrosis, or cholesteatoma. Bone changes are prominent in the mastoid with initial destruction, followed by osteoneogenesis, resulting in dense, sclerotic bone formation. Patients with long-standing COM may also develop hyperostosis of the ossicles, especially the stapes.

Treatment

Medical management usually consists of routine cleaning and topical solutions containing one or more antibiotic and possibly corticosteroids. Systemic antibiotics may also be given for COM. Surgery is usually recommended only if medical therapy fails. Surgery may consist of tympanostomy tube placement if there is insufficient middle ear ventilation, or adenoidectomy if reflux of nasopharyngeal organisms, resulting in middle ear infection, is the problem. Both conditions often coexist, necessitating a combined procedure.

Imaging Findings

CT

Dependent middle ear opacification in two perpendicular planes is characteristic of middle ear effusion, although the characteristics of the fluid (serous, mucous, purulent) cannot be distinguished. Granulation tissue appears as a nondependent middle ear soft tissue opacity with no ossicular displacement or bone erosion. Granulation tissue can also cause nonspecific mastoid opacification. A middle ear cholesterol granuloma can be a complication of COM and is thought to result from eustachian tube dysfunction with secondary mucosal edema and blood vessel rupture. With only middle ear involvement, cholesterol granulomas are generally not associated with bone destruction or erosion and appear on computed tomography (CT) as a nondependent middle ear opacity.

Tympanic membrane abnormalities associated with COM include thickening, calcification, and retractions. Retractions are easily visible on CT and may involve the pars flaccida or pars tensa. Pars flaccida retractions may lead to the development of an acquired cholesteatoma, which is discussed in a separate chapter.

Ossicular erosions can occur with COM in the absence of a cholesteatoma, most likely related to the action of osteoclasts and histiocytes. The most commonly affected areas are the long and lenticular processes of the incus followed by the crura of the stapes, and manubrium of the malleus. Less frequently erosions involve the malleus head and incus body. Widening of the incudostapedial joint in the setting of COM is suspicious for erosion in this region with replacement by fibrous tissue. All of these changes can result in a conductive hearing deficit (CHD).

Ossicular fixation as a consequence of COM can also cause a CHD. Such fixation is the result of the healing process as granulation tissue regresses and fibroblastic invasion of the submucosa develops and adhesions form. This process may take three forms: fibrous tissue fixation, hyalinization of collagen, and fibro-osseous sclerosis. Deposition of fibrous tissue may be focal or generalized and appears as nondependent soft tissue opacification. A common site of involvement is the anterior superior oval window (peristapedial) with stapes fixation. Involvement of the Prussak space results in fixation of the malleus head and neck and can mimic an early cholesteatoma. Involvement of the round window with release of toxins may lead to sensorineural hearing loss (SNHL). Hyalinization of collagen in the middle ear results in tympanosclerosis and is evident on CT as punctate or weblike calcifications in the tympanic cavity, along the tympanic membrane or on ligaments and tendons of the ossicles. Finally fibro-osseous sclerosis results in new bone formation, most commonly in the epitympanum. This appears on CT as a dense bone mass often encasing the ossicles (**Fig. 20–1, Fig. 20–2,** and **Fig. 20–3**).

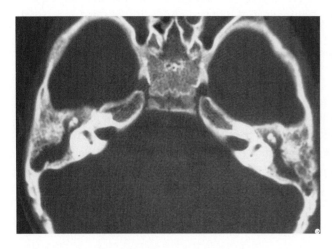

Figure 20–1 Axial computed tomography (CT) of the temporal bones was obtained in a patient with long-standing chronic otitis media. There is mucosal thickening involving both middle ear cavities that is associated with poorly pneumatized and sclerotic mastoid air cells. The sclerosis is likely due to a reactive hyperostosis due to the chronic inflammation.

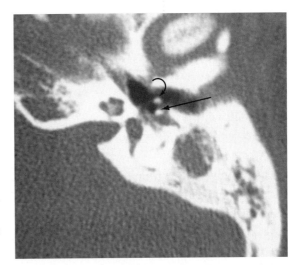

Figure 20–2 Axial CT obtained through the left temporal bone performed in a patient with chronic otitis media shows mucosal thickening surrounding the long process of the incus. The long-standing chronic inflammatory process has resulted in reactive sclerosis of the long process of the incus (*straight arrow*). Note the normal attenuation of the manubrium of the malleus (*curved arrow*). In addition, there is diffuse sclerosis of poorly pneumatized mastoid air cells.

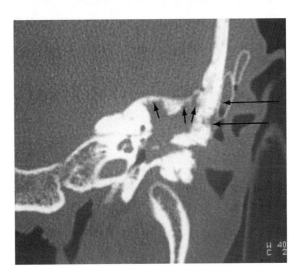

Figure 20–3 Coronal CT performed in a patient with chronic otitis media shows diffuse mucosal thickening, which has scalloped and remodeled that mastoid air cells (*small arrows*). Note the adjacent sclerosis of the surrounding bone (*large arrows*), which is due to the long-standing chronic process. In this case, the findings were due to coalescent mastoiditis but similar findings may also be seen with cholesteatoma.

MRI

Magnetic resonance imaging (MRI), although not helpful in assessing the osseous structures of the middle ear, may be helpful in determining the etiology of soft tissue opacification seen on CT. Middle ear effusions have typical fluid signal on T1- and T2-weighted images with no enhancement. Granulation tissue may have a similar appearance on T1- and T2-weighted MRI, but usually enhances intensely. A cholesteatoma, however, does not enhance, and, if recurrent, may have high signal on diffusion weighted images. Finally, a cholesterol granuloma of the middle ear is hyperintense on T1- and T2-weighted images.

Intracranial complications can develop with COM, similar to those discussed in the chapter on acute otomastoiditis, and are generally best assessed with MRI.

PEARLS _____

- Middle ear effusions or nonspecific opacification are common findings with COM. Nondependent opacification may be secondary to granulation tissue, cholesterol granuloma, cholesteatoma, or fibrous tissue.
- Ossicular erosions can result from COM in the absence of cholesteatoma formation.
- Ossicular fixation may appear as a soft tissue, calcific or osseous mass in the middle ear.

- MRI may be helpful in differentiating the cause of nondependent middle ear opacification seen on CT.
- Intracranial complications are better assessed with MRI.

Suggested Readings

Brook I. Microbiology and management of chronic suppurative otitis media in children. J Trop Pediatr 2003;49:196–199

Canalis RF, Lambert PR. Chronic otitis media and cholesteatoma. In: Canalis RF, Lambert PR, eds. The Ear: Comprehensive Otology. Philadelphia: Lippincott Williams & Wilkins, 2000:409–431

Gates GA. Otitis media with effusion. In: Hughes GB, Pensak ML, eds. Clinical Otology, 2nd ed. New York: Thieme, 1997:205–214

Maheshwari S, Mukherji SK. Diffusion-weighted imaging for differentiating recurrent cholesteatoma from granulation tissue after mastoidectomy: case report. AJNR Am J Neuroradiol 2002;23:847–849

Maroldi R, Farina D, Palvarini A, et al. Computed tomography and magnetic resonance imaging of pathologic conditions of the middle ear. Eur J Radiol 2001;40:78–93

Nemzek WR, Swartz JD. Temporal bone: inflammatory disease. In: Som PM, Curtin HD, eds. Head and Neck Imaging, 4th ed. St. Louis: Mosby, 2003:1173–1229

Swartz JD, Harnsberger HR. The middle ear and mastoid. Imaging of the Temporal Bone, 3rd ed. New York: Thieme, 1998:47–169

CHAPTER 21 Acquired Cholesteatoma

Ellen G. Hoeffner

Epidemiology

Most acquired cholesteatomas result from complications of chronic middle ear infections. Loss of collagen fibers and structural support of the tympanic membrane along with negative middle ear pressure results in a retraction pocket lined with squamous epithelium. Continued negative middle ear pressure and accumulation of epithelial cells, keratin, and cellular decay expand the pocket. Bone destruction of the tympanum and ossicles ensues secondary to direct pressure from the expanding cholesteatoma, biochemical factors related to chronic inflammation and the cholesteatoma itself, and osteoclastic activity. Most cholesteatomas involve the weaker pars flaccida with less common involvement of the pars tensa.

Other potential etiologies of cholesteatoma formation include epithelial invasion through a tympanic membrane perforation, squamous metaplasia of middle ear epithelium, and basal cell hyperplasia.

Clinical Features

Otorrhea and a conductive hearing loss are the most common complaints associated with a cholesteatoma. Patients often have a history of multiple earaches in childhood followed by chronic ear problems. Physical exam demonstrates retraction of the eardrum, often with a perforation, and surrounding bony erosion. Patients with ossicular erosion typically present with a 30- to 60-dB conductive hearing loss. On otoscopic examination, the characteristic clinical finding is the presence of a "pearly white mass" behind the tympanic membrane. However, the tympanic membrane often becomes scarred and retracted in chronic inflammation and the otologist may not be able to accurately assess the middle ear cavity.

Pathology

Cholesteatomas are lined by stratified squamous epithelium and contain desquamated keratin and purulent material.

Treatment

Surgical excision or exteriorization is the treatment of choice. In patients who cannot tolerate surgery, disease can be controlled with repeated cleansing under a surgical microscope.

Imaging Findings

CT

Computed tomography (CT) is the preferred modality when imaging cholesteatomas, as the defining feature is bone destruction. Cholesteatomas typically present as a nondependent middle ear soft tissue mass in a characteristic location associated with bone and ossicular erosion.

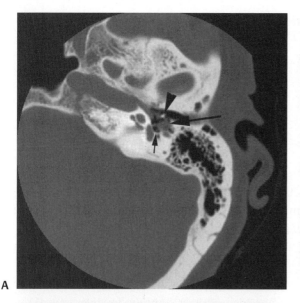
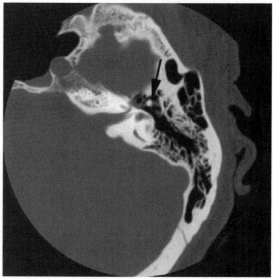

A

B

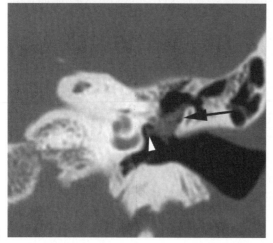

C

Figure 21–1 Computed tomography (CT) findings of choles-teatoma. **(A)** Axial image shows a focal soft tissue mass located within the middle ear cavity (*large arrow*). The manubrium of the malleus (*arrowhead*) and stapes (*small arrow*) are intact. However, the long process of the incus is absent, indicating that it is eroded. These findings are characteristic of a cholesteatoma. **(B)** Axial CT obtained at the level of the epitympanum shows the head of the malleus (*arrow*) is intact but the short process of the incus is absent. **(C)** Coronal CT shows a focal soft tissue mass in the middle ear cavity that extends superiorly into the epitympanum (*large arrow*). The mass extends medially to the capitulum of the stapes (*arrowhead*).

The Prussak space is the site of origin of the more common pars flaccida cholesteatomas, displacing the malleus head and incus body medially and eroding the scutum. The mass can expand into the epitympanum and eventually the antrum and mastoid air cells via the aditus ad antrum, which is often widened by the cholesteatoma.

Less common pars tensa cholesteatomas typically involve the facial recess and sinus tympani of the posterior tympanum. The malleus head and incus body are displaced laterally as these masses extend into the attic. These cholesteatomas also grow medially and can destroy the otic capsule, resulting in a labyrinthine fistula, most commonly involving the lateral semicircular canal.

Other important features to evaluate on CT include involvement of the facial nerve, dehiscence of the tegmen tympani, sigmoid sinus plate destruction, degree of cellularity or sclerosis of the mastoid, level of the dura laterally, and any prior postoperative changes (**Fig. 21–1**).

MRI

Due to its inability to visualize fine bony detail, magnetic resonance imaging (MRI) is more limited in the evaluation of cholesteatomas compared with CT. One area where MRI excels, however, is distinguishing granulation tissue from cholesteatoma. Both of these entities appear similar on CT; however, granulation tissue enhances on MRI whereas a cholesteatoma does not. Diffusion-weighted imaging

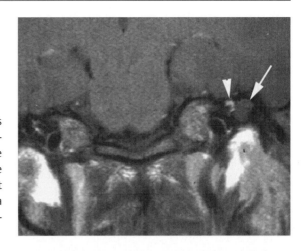

Figure 21–2 Magnetic resonance imaging (MRI) findings of cholesteatoma. Coronal contrast-enhanced MRI demonstrates a nonenhancing focal soft tissue mass located in the left middle ear cavity (*arrow*). Note the enhancement of the tympanic portion of the facial nerve (*arrowhead*). The patient had left facial nerve palsy. This was due to the cholesteatoma directly abutting the facial nerve resulting in acute inflammation of the nerve. These findings were confirmed at surgery.

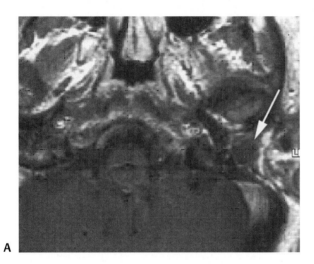

A

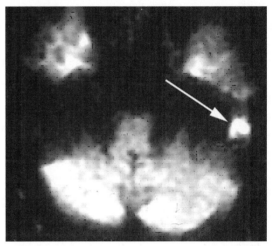

B

Figure 21–3 MRI findings of cholesteatoma. **(A)** Axial contrast-enhanced T1-weighted MRI shows a nonenhancing mass (*arrow*) located in the middle ear cavity in a patient who had undergone two prior ear surgeries and presented with chronic otorrhea, indicative of recurrent cholesteatoma. **(B)** Diffusion-weighted imaging shows the high signal within the mass (*arrow*), also suggestive of recurrent cholesteatoma.

may help differentiate recurrent cholesteatoma from granulation tissue, with the former having high signal on diffusion-weighted images.

Magnetic resonance imaging is also useful in the evaluation of intracranial complications of cholesteatomas such as meningitis, cerebritis, abscess formation, and dural venous sinus thrombosis. In the presence of erosion of the tegmen tympani, MRI can search for a meningocele or meningoencephalocele. With bony involvement of the facial nerve canal or otic capsule, MRI may be helpful in searching for thickening and enhancement of the facial nerve or labyrinth, suggesting inflammation of these structures (**Fig. 21–2** and **Fig. 21–3**).

PEARLS _____

- A nondependent middle ear mass with bone destruction or ossicular erosion on CT is a cholesteatoma 90% of the time. However, only 50% of cholesteatomas have these findings.
- MRI is most helpful in searching for intracranial complications.
- Recurrent cholesteatomas may have high signal on diffusion-weighted images distinguishing them from granulation tissue.

- Other etiologies to be considered in the differential diagnosis of destructive middle ear masses on CT include histiocytosis, giant cell tumor, xanthoma, squamous cell carcinoma, rhabdomyosarcoma, and metastases.

Suggested Readings

Canalis RF, Lambert PR. Chronic otitis media and cholesteatoma. In: Canalis RF, Lambert PR, eds. The Ear: Comprehensive Otology. Philadelphia: Lippincott Williams & Wilkins, 2000:409–431

Chee NWC, Tan TY. The value of pre-operative high resolution CT scans in cholesteatoma surgery. Singapore Med J 2001;42:155–159

Harnsberger HR. Hand Book of Head and Neck Imaging, 2nd ed. St. Louis: Mosby, 1995

Maheshwari S, Mukherji SK. Diffusion-weighted imaging for differentiating recurrent cholesteatoma from granulation tissue after mastoidectomy: case report. AJNR Am J Neuroradiol 2002;23:847–849

Maroldi R, Farina D, Palvarini A, et al. Computed tomography and magnetic resonance imaging of pathologic conditions of the middle ear. Eur J Radiol 2001;40:78–93

Nemzek WR, Swartz JD. Temporal bone: inflammatory disease. In: Som PM, Curtin HD, eds. Head and Neck Imaging, 4th ed. St. Louis: Mosby, 2003:1173–1229

Yates PD, Flood LM, Banerjee A, et al. CT scanning of middle ear cholesteatomas: what does the surgeon want to know? Br J Radiol 2002;75:847–852

CHAPTER 22 Cholesterol Granuloma

Hemant Parmar

Epidemiology

Cholesterol granuloma, also called "cholesterol cyst" and "chocolate ear," is an expansile, inflammatory mass of granulation tissue in the middle ear. The term *cholesterol granuloma* refers to its pathologic features, whereas *cholesterol cyst* describes its gross appearance. It develops as a result of obstruction that leads to a repetitive cycle of hemorrhage and granulation tissue formation. It is a foreign body reaction to cholesterol deposits that occur in obstructed fluid-filled air cells of the temporal bone. It can also occur in the petrous apex and mastoid air cells, but is more common in the middle ear.

There are two theories proposed to describe its occurrence. According to the classic "obstruction-vacuum" hypothesis, cholesterol granulomas form when there is mucosal swelling obstructing the circuitous pneumatic pathway. There is resorption of the gas in obstructed cells, creating relative vacuum and rupture of the blood vessels. Cholesterol granuloma forms from the anaerobic breakdown of the blood products. According to the "exposed marrow" theory, there is obstruction secondary to inflammation. This is due to budding of the mucosa in young adults that invades and replaces the hematopoietic marrow of the temporal bone. Hemorrhage from the exposed marrow coagulates within the mucosal cells and occludes the outflow pathway. This sustained hemorrhage provides the engine for progressive cyst expansion.

Clinical Features

Patients with cholesterol granuloma often have a history of purulent or serous otitis media and allergies. Young and middle-aged adults are usually affected. Distribution is equal for both sexes. Most patients have symptoms running for 2 to 3 years and present with slowly progressive conductive deafness. Unlike cholesterol granulomas of the petrous apex, there are no cranial neuropathies. On examination, there is bluish discoloration of the eardrum ("blue eardrum"). The growth pattern is variable and depends on the frequency of hemorrhages within the lesion over a period of time.

Pathology

Cholesterol cyst contains brownish liquid with cholesterol crystals and brownish sediment. On histopathology cholesterol granuloma consists of numerous clefts of cholesterol crystals surrounded by histiocytes, round cells, macrophages, giant cells, and abnormal fragile blood vessels. These blood vessels are often prone to rupture, resulting in areas of hemorrhage and hemosiderin deposition. Cholesterol granulomas are lined by fibrous connective tissue.

Treatment

Symptomatic cases are treated with surgical resection of the cyst walls and their contents. For recurrent and intractable disease, mastoidectomy may have to be performed.

Imaging Findings

CT

Early and small cholesterol granulomas present as nonspecific soft tissue lesions in the middle ear cavity without any bony or ossicular erosions. Later, with expansion and growth of the cyst they appear as sharply and smoothly marginated lesions causing bony scalloping. The ossicular chain is displaced. The mastoid air cells and middle ear cavity are opacified, often from repeated infections. Magnetic resonance imaging (MRI) shows no enhancement in cholesterol granulomas and is not necessary for diagnosis, unless there is difficulty in distinguishing early granulomas from glomus tumor, which shows marked enhancement. Middle ear cholesterol granuloma should be distinguished from other lesions of the middle ear, such as hemorrhagic otitis media (no bony expansion), cholesteatoma (erosive bone changes with ossicular destruction), paraganglioma (erosive bone changes, intense enhancement with contrast), encephalocele (defect in tegmen tympani), and vascular anomaly like aberrant carotid artery (**Fig. 22–1**).

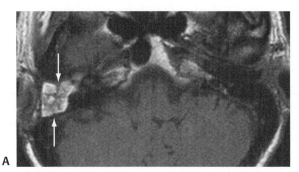
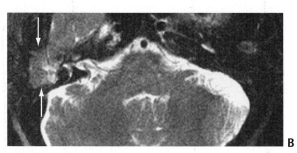

Figure 22–1 (A) Axial noncontrast T1-weighted (T1W) image through the right temporal bone shows a predominantly high signal mass involving the middle ear and right mastoid cavity (*arrows*). **(B)** Axial T2W image shows the mass to be intermediate signal.
(Case courtesy of Vincent Chong, MD, Singapore.)

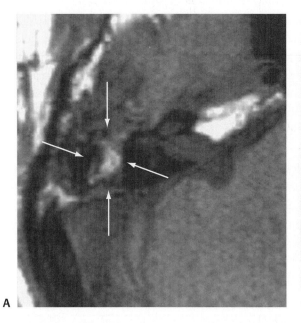
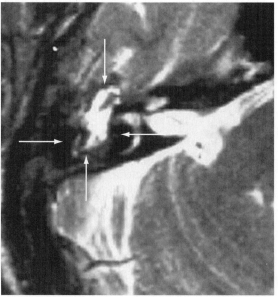

Figure 22–2 (A) Axial noncontrast T1W image through the right temporal bone shows this middle ear cholesterol granuloma to have a much more heterogeneous signal (*arrows*) than the case presented in **Figure 22–1**. **(B)** The Axial T2W image shows this mass to be primarily high signal (*arrows*).
(Case courtesy of Vincent Chong, MD, Singapore.)

MRI

Magnetic resonance imaging (MRI) is complementary to CT in making the diagnosis. On MRI cholesterol granulomas exhibit T1 hyperintensity due to the presence of paramagnetic methemoglobin. The T2-weighted images may show variable signal depending on the protein content, the phase of the blood product (including hemosiderin), and the extent of underlying granulation tissue (**Fig. 22–2**).

PEARLS _____

- CT and MRI are complementary in making the correct diagnosis.
- Expansile mass of the middle ear with smooth and sharp bony margins, often with opacification of the mastoid air cells due to chronic infection.
- The diagnosis can be suggested by the presence of a high T1-weighted signal lesion centered in the middle ear cavity in an adult.

Suggested Readings

Jackler RK, Cho M. A new theory to explain the genesis of petrous apex cholesterol granuloma. Otol Neurotol 2003;24:96–106 discussion 106

Maeta M, Saito R, Nakagawa F, Miyahara T. Surgical intervention in middle-ear cholesterol granuloma. J Laryngol Otol 2003;117:344–348

Martin N, Sterkers O, Mompoint D, Julien N, Nahum H. Cholesterol granulomas of the middle ear cavities: MR imaging. Radiology 1989;172:521–525

Nager G. Pathology of the Ear and Temporal Bone. Baltimore: Williams & Wilkins, 1992

Palacios E, Valvassori G. Petrous apex lesions: cholesterol granuloma. Ear Nose Throat J 1999;78:234

CHAPTER 23 Histiocytosis

Mohannad Ibrahim

Epidemiology

Langerhans cell histiocytosis (LCH) is a rare disease with an incidence of 0.2 to 2.0 cases per 100,000 children under 15 years of age. It comprises a wide spectrum of clinical manifestations associated with the proliferation of Langerhans cells. The term was adopted by the Philadelphia Workshop of the Histiocyte Society to identify a group of diseases previously known as eosinophilic granuloma of bone, Hand-Schüller-Christian disease, and Letterer-Siwe disease. LCH may present as isolated osseous involvement (36%), isolated nonosseous involvement (33%), or multisystem involvement. It can be unifocal (65%) or multifocal (35%). Bony involvement is the most frequent, with estimated 15 to 61% of the patients having otologic involvement, with bilateral temporal involvement seen in 30% of the patients. Children with otologic involvement have a higher risk of poor response and higher percentage of second line treatment.

Clinical Features

Langerhans cell histiocytosis usually presents in the first decade. There is an inverse relationship between age of presentation and severity of disease, with Letterer-Siwe disease present in the first 3 years, Hand-Schüller-Christian present between 3 and 5 years, and unifocal LCH (eosinophilic granuloma) present between 5 and 20 years. Otologic involvement is usually seen in younger age groups and is more frequently seen in multisystemic disease. It can be the initial presentation in 5 to 25% of patients. Patients with temporal bone involvement can infrequently be asymptomatic; however, patients are commonly symptomatic and usually present with chronic otorrhea, mastoiditis, external auditory canal lesions, otitis, and conductive or sensorineural hearing loss. Diagnostic errors are frequent because the otologic findings are similar to those of other conditions, particularly otomastoiditis.

Pathology

Langerhans cell histiocytosis is characterized by proliferation of abnormal histiocytes, which share many structural and immunophenotypic features with Langerhans' cells, with the presence of cytoplasmic inclusion bodies seen in electron microscopy, known as Birbeck granules. Langerhans cell proliferation can involve any tissue or organ in the body, and the clinical picture is heterogeneous. Involvement of the skeletal, cutaneous, lymphoreticular (including liver, spleen, lymph nodes, and bone marrow), pulmonary, and pituitary gland is seen most often.

Treatment

There is a 90% cure rate for unifocal temporal LCH. Surgical curettage or mastoidectomy is often required for mastoid and middle ear disease. Low-dose radiotherapy is used for larger lesions. The prevalence of multisystemic disease in these patients has been shown to have an unfavorable effect on treatment response, and therefore a greater percentage of patients required second-line therapy. Chemotherapy, steroids, and immunotherapy are often required in patients with multisystemic disease.

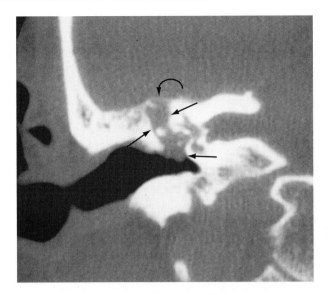

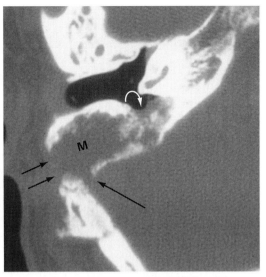

Figure 23–1 Coronal computed tomography (CT) demonstrates an aggressive soft tissue mass involving the middle ear cavity (*straight arrows*). The mass extends superiorly into the epitympanum with early bony destruction of the tegmen tympani (*curved arrow*).

Figure 23–2 Axial CT through the right temporal shows a destructive mass involving the mastoid portion of the temporal bone. The mass extends medially and invades the posterior aspect of the middle ear cavity (*curved arrow*). Posteriorly, there is erosion of the dural sinus plate (*straight long arrow*). The mass extends laterally and erodes the lateral cortex of the temporal bone (*straight short arrows*). Biopsy revealed histiocytosis.

Imaging Findings

CT

Langerhans cell histiocytosis commonly presents as a destructive lesion that involves the mastoid complex and less commonly involves the squamous portion of the temporal bone or the middle ear. Destruction of the middle ear ossicles, isolated petrous apex involvement, or labyrinthine involvement is rare. There is usually an associated soft tissue mass that commonly has homogeneous enhancement and less commonly heterogeneous enhancement. Associated intracranial extradural extension is best seen on postcontrast imaging (**Figs. 23–1** and **Fig. 23–2**).

MRI

The soft tissue mass has variable signal intensity on T1-weighted imaging and is hyperintense on T2-weighted imaging, often with edema or inflammation around the lesion. There is variable enhancement after administration of gadolinium. The radiologic differential diagnosis includes acute otomastoiditis, acquired cholesteatoma, rhabdomyosarcoma, and metastatic disease (**Fig. 23–3**).

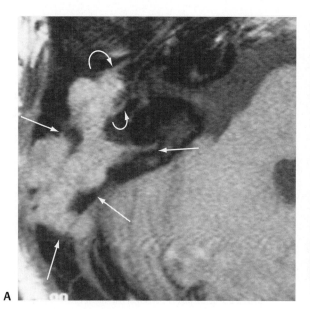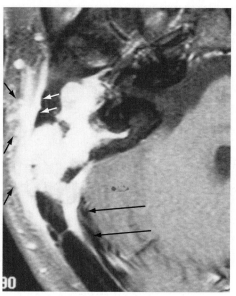

Figure 23–3 (A) Axial noncontrast T1-weighted image shows an intermediate signal mass invading the temporal bone (*straight arrows*) with extension into the middle ear cavity (*curved arrows*). **(B)** The mass densely enhances fol-lowing contrast administration. Note the extension into the soft tissues overlying the temporal bone (*small arrows*) and dural involvement of the posterior fossa (*large arrows*).

PEARLS _____

- Consider LCH when a temporal bone lesion does not respond to antibiotics and a tympanotomy tube.
- The clinical presentation and radiologic findings can be diagnostic of LCH, especially in bilateral involvement; however, a biopsy is usually required for the definitive diagnosis of temporal LCH.

Suggested Readings

Fernández-Latorre F, Menor-Serrano F, Alonso-Charterina S, Arenas-Jiménez J. Langerhans cell his-tiocytosis of the temporal bone in pediatric patients: imaging and follow-up. AJR Am J Roentgenol 2000;174:217–221

Howarth DM, Gilchrist GS, Mullan BP, Wiseman GA, Edmonson JH, Schomberg PJ. Langerhans Cell Histiocytosis: Diagnosis, Natural History, Management, and Outcome. American Cancer Society 1999:2278–2290

McCaffrey TV, McDonald TJ. Histiocytosis X of the ear and temporal bone: review of 22 cases. Laryngo-scope 1979;89:1735–1742

Prayer D, Grois N, Prosch H, Gadner H, Barkovich AJ. MR imaging presentation of intracranial disease associated with Langerhans cell histiocytosis. AJNR Am J Neuroradiol 2004;25:880–891

Surico G, Muggeo P, Muggeo V, et al. Ear involvement in childhood Langerhans cell histiocytosis. Head Neck 2000;22:42–47

CHAPTER 24 Paraganglioma

Douglas J. Quint

Epidemiology

Temporal bone paragangliomas/chemodectomas are most commonly found along cranial nerves IX and X. Within the temporal bone region, they occur in the middle ear cleft on the cochlear promontory (20%) or the hypotympanum (25%) as glomus tympanicum tumors, the jugular foramen region (50%) as glomus jugulare tumors, or just below the skull base (5%) as glomus vagale tumors. Lesions involving the middle ear and jugular fossa regions are called glomus jugulotympanicum tumors. Paragangliomas are the most common primary middle ear neoplasm.

The incidence of temporal bone paragangliomas is approximately 1/million/year, and somewhat preferentially occur in middle-aged women.

When spontaneously occurring, these lesions are multiple in 5 to 10% of patients, but are multiple in up to 50% of patients in familial cases.

Clinical Features

Presenting symptoms in patients with these neoplasm are a function of the location of the tumor. Middle ear lesions (glomus tympanicum tumors) can present with pulsatile tinnitus (80 to 90%) as they are vascular tumors, conductive hearing loss (50 to 60%) as ossicles can be affected, otalgia, or simply a sense of ear "fullness." Less than 5% of these tumors are physiologically active, producing catecholamines (norepinephrine). Middle ear paragangliomas are essentially never physiologically active. On physical examination, these lesions can be seen as a reddish vascular mass behind the anteroinferior portion of the tympanic membrane.

Pathology

All paragangliomas/chemodectomas, regardless of location, are histologically identical. They arise from embryonic neural crest cells that have differentiated into paraganglia (chemoreceptor cells). These extremely vascular, but histologically benign tumors are composed of central "chief" cells that are arranged in a typical pattern called "zellballen." Less than 5% of these "chief" cells actively secrete catecholamines. More aggressive tumor variants can have similar histology but can only be diagnosed when metastatic lesions are present (<5% of patients).

Treatment

Preoperative endovascular embolization, surgery, or radiation therapy are potential therapies for larger lesions. Smaller lesions (which include essentially all lesions confined to the middle ear region) are usually treated with surgery only. Complete resection is curative.

Imaging Findings

When tumors are large, their respective site of origin can be obscure, as the jugular foramen, middle ear, and petrous temporal bone regions may all be involved. Such large tumors of the temporal bone may simply be referred to as glomus jugulotympanicum tumors and should be characterized with computed tomography (CT) (osseous involvement) and magnetic resonance imaging (MRI) (intracranial and infratemporal extension; differentiating tumor from trapped middle ear or mastoid secretions). When confined to the middle ear cleft, these tumors can arise anywhere on the medial wall of the mesotympanum and hypotympanum (i.e., along the course of the tympanic branch of cranial nerve IX), not just the cochlear promontory region, and are considered glomus tympanicum tumors. Such smaller tumors can be adequately characterized with CT without the need for MRI.

CT

High-resolution (1 to 2 mm) noncontrast CT performed in the axial and coronal planes and reconstructed with a detail (bone) algorithm best delineates temporal bone structures. Sagittal reformatted images may also prove useful.

On CT scans, because of the superior spatial resolution, a small middle ear paraganglioma is best localized and delineated. CT is the only imaging modality necessary to search for small tumors on the cochlear promontory or involving only the hypotympanic region. Glomus jugulare or glomus jugulotympanicum tumors can enlarge the jugular foramen, erode the jugular spine, or destroy the osseous margin between the jugular foramen and the carotid canal. These lesions can frankly invade and destroy portions of the temporal bone. The extent of osseous destruction is best characterized with multiplanar CT (**Fig. 24–1A**).

There is no role for contrast-enhanced CT imaging in these patients.

MRI

Thin-section multiplanar pre- and postcontrast T1- and T2-weighted scanning is best for delineating the overall extent of lesions, particularly when they invade the temporal bone or extend intracranially or below the temporal bone (**Fig. 24–1B, Fig. 24–2A,** and **Fig. 24–2B**).

Magnetic resonance is excellent for showing the typical "salt and pepper" (flow voids) appearance of paragangliomas (on noncontrast T1-weighted scan) when such lesions are large (usual presentation for glomus vagale, jugulare, and carotid paragangliomas), but such flow voids will not be seen in small middle ear lesions (glomus tympanicum paraganglioma). Paragangliomas demonstrate intermediate heterogeneous signal on T2-weighted scans. As these lesions are quite vascular, they enhance on contrast-enhanced T1-weighted scans. Even very small temporal bone lesions can be detected on contrast-enhanced MRI scans. However, when definitively identified as a small medial wall middle ear lesion on CT without associated osseous destruction, additional MRI is not necessary.

When a larger lesion is associated with opacification of the middle ear and mastoid regions, MRI can differentiate tumor from trapped secretions. Contrast-enhanced MRI can enhance the glomus tumor, whereas contiguous trapped secretions do not enhance. Similarly, on T2-weighted scans, trapped secretions are hyperintense, whereas glomus tumors are heterogeneously isointense to brain (**Fig. 24–2B**).

Other Imaging

Endovascular angiography can be performed for larger lesions so that the extent of these highly vascular tumors can be assessed and preoperative embolization performed as necessary. These lesions are supplied by internal or external carotid branches depending on their locations (**Fig. 24–2C**). MRI angiography is of no value when evaluating these lesions. Smaller, typical appearing purely mesotympanic paragangliomas do not require preoperative angiography.

Indium scintigraphy has been used to identify somatostatin receptors in paragangliomas, but the sensitivity of this technique for small lesions in the temporal bones remains unknown.

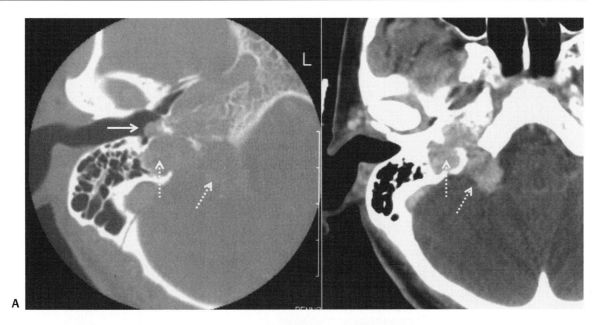

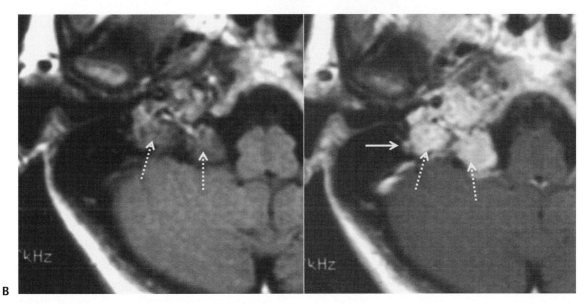

Figure 24-1 A 49-year-old woman presents with right-sided pulsatile tinnitus, dizziness, loss of balance, and headache. **(A)** Axial contrast-enhanced bone window (left) and brain window (right) computed tomography (CT) scans through the right skull base demonstrate the enhancing mass involving the right cerebellomedullary cistern and the right jugular foramen region (*dotted arrows*), but better demonstrate the MRI (**Fig. 24-1B**) associated osseous destruction and the right middle ear involvement (*solid arrow*). Angiography confirmed the presence of a vascular glomus jugulotympanicum tumor, which encased the right internal carotid artery at the skull base. The patient failed a balloon test occlusion and was treated with radiation therapy with resolution of symptoms.

(B) Axial precontrast (left) and contrast-enhanced (right) T1-weighted magnetic resonance imaging (MRI) through the right skull base region demonstrates the enhancing mass involving the right cerebellomedullary cistern and the right jugular foramen region (*dotted arrows*) with minimal extension into the right middle ear cleft (*solid arrow*).

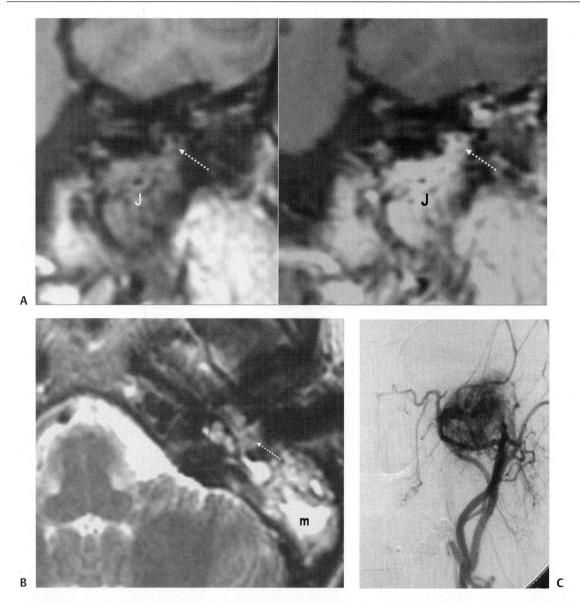

Figure 24–2 A 37-year-old woman with a history of pulsatile tinnitus on the left for 2 years, 6 months of progressive left-sided hearing loss and recent otitis media. **(A)** Coronal pre-contrast (left) and contrast-enhanced (right) T1-weighted MRI through the left skull base region demonstrates an enhancing jugular foramen mass (J) with cephalad extension into the temporal bone and left middle ear region (*dotted arrows*). **(B)** Axial T2-weighted MRI through the left temporal bone demonstrates the middle ear portion of the mass (*dot-*ted arrow*) isointense to brain. Trapped mastoid secretions (m) demonstrate increased signal on this T2-weighted study. Note: Temporal bone tumor is easily delineated from contiguous trapped secretions on the T2-weighted MRI scans. Such differentiation is impossible on CT and can be difficult on T1-weighted MRI scans. **(C)** Anteroposterior left carotid angiography demonstrates the highly vascular nature of this subsequently resected jugulotympanicum tumor.

Differential Diagnosis

Vascular anomalies such as an aberrant (laterally located) intratemporal course of the internal carotid artery, a dehiscent jugular bulb, or a persistent stapedial artery can usually be inferred by careful inspection of a skull base CT as the osseous structures that usually delineate these vascular structures will not be normal. As necessary, magnetic resonance angiography (MRA) or even endovascular angiography may be necessary to sort out anomalous vasculature.

A *congenital* (primary) *cholesteatoma* is usually seen in children or teenagers, is a whitish (not reddish) retrotympanic mass clinically, and does not enhance on contrast-enhanced imaging.

Other tumors such as *schwannomas* and *hemangiomas* can be seen in the middle ear region, but both are usually more closely related to cranial nerve VII. Aggressive tumors are rare in the middle ear region, but include adenocarcinoma, squamous cell carcinoma, sarcoma, and metastatic disease.

PEARLS

- These lesions can be aggressive and can invade the temporal bone, the carotid space of the suprahyoid neck, or the intracranial region. When large, their site of origin (e.g., middle ear, jugular foramen) can be impossible to determine.
- Purely middle ear lesions can be evaluated with only noncontrast CT scanning. For larger lesions, both CT and MRI and sometimes angiography are necessary.
- One must differentiate a purely middle ear lesion (glomus tympanicum) from a lesion that also involves the jugular foramen region (glomus jugulotympanicum) because the surgical approach is different. Surgery for glomus jugulotympanicum tumors is a more complicated operation.

Suggested Readings

Harnsberger HR, ed. Diagnostic Imaging: Head and Neck. Salt Lake City: Amirsys, 2004

Noujaim SE, Pattekar MA, Cacciarelli A, Sanders WP, Wang AM. Paraganglioma of the temporal bone: role of magnetic resonance imaging versus computed tomography. Top Magn Reson Imaging 2000;11:108–122

Pellitteri PK, Rinaldo A, Myssiorek D, et al. Paragangliomas of the head and neck. Oral Oncol 2004;40: 563–575

Saringer W, Kitz K, Czerny C, et al. Paragangliomas of the temporal bone: results of different treatment modalities in 53 patients. Acta Neurochir (Wien) 2002;144:1255–1264

Swartz JD, Harnsberger HR, eds. Imaging of the Temporal Bone, 3rd ed. New York: Thieme, 1998

Weissman JL, Hirsch BE. Beyond the promontory: the multifocal origin of glomus tympanicum tumors. AJNR Am J Neuroradiol 1998;19:119–122

CHAPTER 25 Schwannoma
Douglas J. Quint

Epidemiology

Facial nerve schwannomas are found in 5% of all patients who present with a facial nerve palsy. Although facial nerve schwannomas can arise anywhere along the facial nerve from the brainstem to the parotid gland, the most commonly involved portions of the nerve are within the temporal bone, specifically the geniculate, tympanic, second genu (region of facial nerve recess), and mastoid regions. Along with hemangiomas, schwannomas are the most common tumors of the facial nerve canal; 0.8% of all petrous temporal bone tumors are schwannomas. Intratemporal facial nerve schwannomas are more common than internal auditory canal facial nerve schwannomas. Less than 10% of seventh nerve schwannomas arise in the parotid gland. These tumors can arise in patients of any age, although the age range of 30 to 40 years is most commonly affected.

Clinical Features

Presenting symptoms depend on the location of the lesion. When arising within the temporal bone, facial nerve dysfunction (e.g., palsy) due to compression of the facial nerve is usually seen (50 to 90% of patients). When occurring as a tympanic cavity lesion (which is the most frequent location for these tumors), they can erode the ossicles resulting in conductive hearing loss (60 to 70% of patients). Symptom onset is usually gradual, but rarely can be acute and even intermittent. When lesions arise in the internal auditory canal, patients may present with sensorineural hearing loss with or without facial nerve dysfunction. Intraparotid seventh nerve schwannomas do not compress the facial nerve and present as an asymptomatic parotid mass.

Pathology

Facial nerve schwannomas, like schwannomas elsewhere, are benign peripheral nervous system tumors arising from the perineural lining cells—the nerve sheath (Schwann) cells. Histologically, regions of Antoni A (more cellularity) and Antoni B (less cellularity) tissue are seen. Tumors usually extend away from the nerve, which is why they are asymptomatic when arising in the soft parotid gland. However, in the confining intratemporal facial nerve canal, even when these tumors are small, symptomatic compression of the facial nerve can occur.

Treatment

Due to risks of injuring the facial nerve and the benign nature of these tumors, conservative therapy with serial imaging is the usual management with decompressive surgery (resection of tumor with nerve grafting as necessary) reserved for those who develop higher grade facial paralyses.

Imaging Findings

As these lesions can involve any portion of the facial nerve, the entire intratemporal facial nerve must be evaluated. Computed tomography (CT) is best for assessing the morphology of the facial nerve canal and any associated canal or ossicular erosion or frank destruction. Magnetic resonance imaging (MRI) is best for directly demonstrating the tumor, particularly its true extent along the facial nerve including portions where there has not yet been erosion of the facial nerve canal. Internal auditory canal (IAC) involvement, cerebellopontine angle (CPA) cistern involvement, intracranial extension (into the middle cranial fossa via the greater superficial petrosal nerve), and infratemporal (e.g., parotid) extension is also best assessed with MRI.

CT

High-resolution (1 to 2 mm) noncontrast CT performed in the axial and coronal planes and reconstructed with a detail (bone) algorithm best delineates the facial nerve canal. Sagittal reformatted images are also sometimes useful, particularly when evaluating the mastoid portion of the facial canal.

A lesion may only manifest as a subtle mass along a portion of the intratemporal course of the seventh nerve. Specifically, the facial nerve canal should be assessed for smoothly marginated, well-defined canal enlargement with special attention to geniculate fossa, and also to the labyrinthine, tympanic, and mastoid portions of the canal (**Fig. 25–1**). Also, a search for a mass in the middle ear cleft arising from the region of the geniculate ganglion or the tympanic portion of the seventh nerve with or without associated erosion of contiguous middle and inner ear structures should be performed. Rare extension by a lesion beyond the temporal bone can be suggested by temporal bone destruction.

There is no role for contrast-enhanced CT imaging in these patients.

MRI

Thin-section multiplanar pre- and postcontrast T1- and T2-weighted scanning is best for delineating the overall extent of lesions, particularly when they do not enlarge the facial nerve canal. Schwannomas are relatively vascular lesions that demonstrate contrast-enhancement.

Facial nerve schwannomas demonstrate low T1 signal, increased T2 signal, and homogeneous contrast enhancement. The entire course of the seventh nerve (CPA, IAC, intratemporal, parotid) should be assessed. Even when a focal enhancing lesion consistent with a schwannoma is found, one needs to check for enhancement of contiguous, nonenlarged facial nerve that may represent a tumor "tail" because these lesions can extend for centimeters.

Magnetic resonance and CT imaging are complementary. In the setting of a positive MRI scan, a CT scan to better delineate osseous involvement is still often of value.

Differential Diagnosis

Normal perivascular enhancement by normal vascular structures is usually seen in the geniculate and proximal horizontal (tympanic) portions of the seventh nerve canal. Such findings are symmetric, and are not associated with mass effect or osseous changes.

A *facial nerve hemangioma* can be impossible to differentiate from a facial nerve schwannoma when the lesions are located in the geniculate ganglion region. However, hemangiomas tend to be more focal, less well defined, will not have an enhancing "tail" extending along the facial nerve, and can have spiculated osseous involvement ("ossifying hemangioma") on CT.

A *viral neuritis (Bell palsy)* can demonstrate enhancement of a portion of the seventh nerve, which may or may not involve the geniculate region. Such an infectious process is not associated with osseous changes and does not expand or destroy the facial nerve canal. Unlike a schwannoma, the neural enhancement often resolves over months.

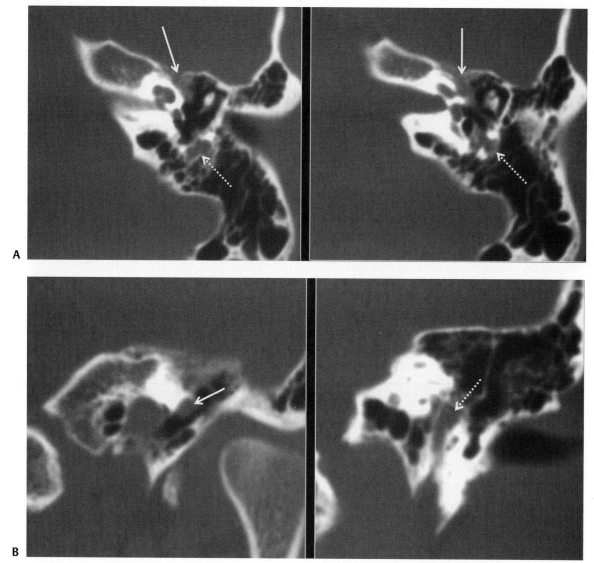

Figure 25–1 A 16-year-old boy with progressive left facial nerve paralysis developing over 6 months. **(A)** Axial noncontrast computed tomography (CT) scans through the left temporal bone demonstrates a mass centered in the region of the geniculate ganglion (*solid arrow*) extending posteriorly into the proximal horizontal (tympanic) portion of the seventh nerve canal. A second lesion is seen in the facial nerve recess (second genu of the seventh cranial nerve) region (*dotted arrow*).

(B) Coronal noncontrast CT scans through the left temporal bone (anterior on the left; more posterior on the right) demonstrates the enlargement of the proximal tympanic segment of the facial nerve canal (*solid arrow*) and the enlargement of the second genu and proximal descending portion of the facial nerve canal (*dotted arrow*). Decompressive surgery demonstrated facial nerve schwannomas in both regions of facial nerve canal enlargement.

A *congenital cholesteatoma* has well-defined osseous margins, but most importantly does not demonstrate enhancement on contrast-enhanced MRI.

An *acquired cholesteatoma* usually arises in the lateral aspect of the middle ear cleft and presents with a different clinical story. Depending on the degree of inflammation, these lesions can enhance.

Perineural spread by neoplasm tends to occur when carcinomas (squamous cell, adenoid cystic) extend through the skull base, and therefore typically involves the more distal portions of the facial nerve canal. However, such lesions can mimic facial nerve schwannomas. Often there is a history of previously treated parotid or skull base neoplasm. Imaging studies should be reviewed for contiguous primary neoplasms.

PEARLS _____

- On a noncontrast temporal bone CT, search for enlargement of any portion of the facial nerve canal, with special attention to the geniculate fossa. Search for extension into middle cranial fossa, IAC, or below the skull base. Search for ossicular erosion (patient presents with conductive hearing loss) or inner ear involvement (that could result in fistulas at surgery).
- On a contrast-enhanced MRI scan, all lesions should enhance. Assess the entire intracranial, temporal bone, and parotid course of the seventh cranial nerve. Search for enhancement of nonenlarged portions of the facial nerve contiguous with bulkier tumor to define the true extent of a lesion.

Suggested Readings

Chung SY, Kim DI, Lee BH, Yoon PH, Jeon P, Chung TS. Facial nerve schwannomas: CT and MR findings. Yonsei Med J 1998;39:148–153

Gebarski SS, Telian SA, Niparko JK. Enhancement along the normal facial nerve in the facial canal: MR imaging and anatomic correlation. Radiology 1992;183:391–394

Harnsberger HR, ed. Diagnostic Imaging: Head and Neck. Salt Lake City: Amirsys, 2004

Jager L, Reiser M. CT and MR imaging of the normal and pathologic conditions of the facial nerve. Eur J Radiol 2001;40:133–136

Kim C-S, Chang SO, Oh SH, Ahn S-H, Hwang CH, Lee HJ. Management of intratemporal facial nerve schwannoma. Otol Neurotol 2003;24:312–316

Michel O, Wagner M, Guntinas-Lichius O. Schwannoma of the greater superficial petrosal nerve. Otolaryngol Head Neck Surg 2000;122:302–303

Swartz JD, Harnsberger HR, eds. Imaging of the Temporal Bone, 3rd ed. New York: Thieme, 1998

CHAPTER 26 Hemangioma
Douglas J. Quint

Epidemiology

Along with schwannomas, hemangiomas are the most common tumors of the facial nerve canal; 0.7% of all petrous temporal bone tumors are hemangiomas. They can occur at any age, but usually are found in adults. Within the temporal bone, the most common location of a hemangioma is the geniculate fossa (region of first genu of the facial nerve canal in the region of the geniculate ganglion), with the internal auditory canal being a less common location for these tumors. Rarely are hemangiomas found in the second genu (facial nerve recess) region.

Clinical Features

As this lesion arises from perineural (facial nerve) vasculature, it is not surprising that it usually presents with facial nerve dysfunction. Symptoms may be due to nerve compression or frank invasion. Symptom onset may be relatively acute (arising over weeks) or more insidious. Symptoms are dependent on the location of the lesion; geniculate fossa lesions present with isolated facial nerve dysfunction, whereas internal auditory canal lesions present with both facial nerve dysfunction and sensorineural hearing loss due to the proximity of the vestibulocochlear (eighth cranial) nerve to the facial nerve in the internal auditory canal.

Pathology

Hemangiomas are slow-growing benign vascular tumors arising from perineural vessels that surround the intratemporal facial nerve. As these vessels appear to be most numerous along the geniculate and proximal tympanic portions of the facial nerve, it is not surprising that those locations are where hemangiomas most commonly occur. Hemangiomas may be divided into three histologic subtypes: (1) ossifying hemangioma (associated with spicules of lamellar bone), (2) cavernous hemangioma (associated with large vascular channels), and (3) capillary hemangioma (associated with small vascular channels). It should be noted that all three histologic subtypes may be present in a single lesion. Hemangiomas can cause symptoms both by nerve compression and invasion. They can invade the nerve (even when lesions are quite small), requiring resection of that part of the nerve for definitive treatment.

Treatment

Complete surgical resection of a hemangioma is curative. No chemotherapy or radiation therapy is necessary. When a lesion is small, it may still be extraneural (causing symptoms by nerve compression only) and the lesion may be completely resected with preservation of seventh nerve function. However, whether large or small, if the lesion has invaded the seventh nerve, that portion of the nerve along with the hemangioma may need to be resected with placement of a nerve graft. Such patients who require grafting have greater morbidity than those who undergo nerve-sparing procedures.

Imaging Findings

Lesions usually present when they are small (<1 cm in size) as they either invade the facial nerve or compress the nerve within the facial nerve canal. Therefore, computed tomography (CT), which can delineate more subtle osseous changes and also demonstrate the typical appearance of ossifying hemangiomas, is the first examination of choice in those patients who present with isolated seventh nerve palsy. For patients who present with seventh nerve palsy and sensorineural/mixed hearing loss, magnetic resonance imaging (MRI) to assess the internal auditory canal is the initial examination of choice.

CT

High-resolution (1 to 2 mm) noncontrast CT performed in the axial and coronal planes and reconstructed with a "detail" (bone) algorithm best delineates the facial nerve canal. As capillary/cavernous hemangiomas can remodel the canal (e.g., in the geniculate region) or enlarge the internal auditory canal, these areas should be carefully examined for abnormality. However, a lesion may only manifest as a subtle mass along the course of the intratemporal portion of the seventh nerve. Ossifying hemangiomas have a somewhat unique appearance as they invade bone, have ill-defined margins, and demonstrate a "honeycomb" appearance of those portions of the petrous temporal bone (in the region of geniculate portion of seventh nerve) that they invade. There is no role for contrast-enhanced CT imaging in these patients (**Fig. 26–1** and **Fig. 26–2**).

MRI

Thin-section multiplanar pre- and postcontrast T1- and T2-weighted scanning is best for delineating the overall extent of lesions, particularly when they do not enlarge the facial nerve canal. This is because hemangiomas are vascular lesions that demonstrate intense contrast enhancement.

Cavernous/capillary hemangiomas have intermediate signal on noncontrast T1-weighted scans, enhance intensely (**Fig. 26–1B** and **Fig. 26–2A**), and demonstrate heterogeneous, but predominantly increased, signal on T2 weighted scans. Ossifying hemangiomas demonstrate ill-defined margins and heterogeneous T1 and T2 signal in the region of their osseous involvement. They also enhance intensely.

Differential Diagnosis (Geniculate Hemangiomas)

Normal perivascular enhancement by normal vascular structures is usually seen in the geniculate and proximal horizontal (tympanic) portions of the seventh nerve canal. Such findings are symmetric, and are not associated with mass effect or osseous changes.

A *facial nerve schwannoma* can be impossible to differentiate from capillary/cavernous hemangiomas. However, schwannomas are often larger lesions (greater than 1 cm) at presentation.

A *viral neuritis (Bell palsy)* can demonstrate enhancement of a portion of the seventh nerve, which may or may not involve the geniculate region. Such an infectious process is not associated with osseous changes and does not expand or destroy the facial nerve canal. Unlike a hemangioma, the neural enhancement often resolves over months.

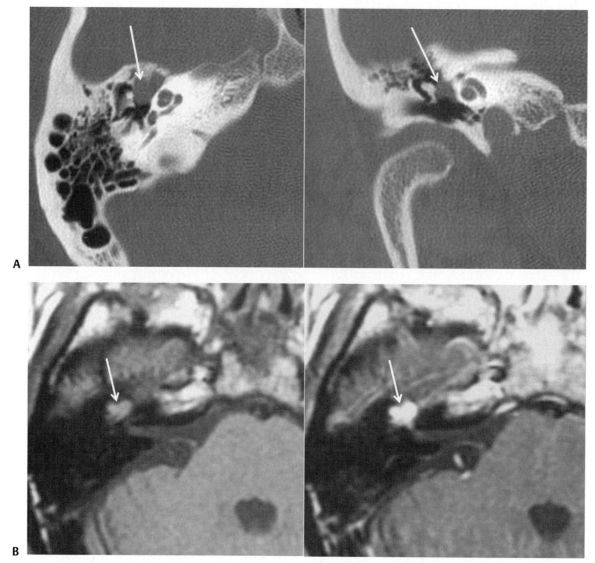

Figure 26–1 A 49-year-old man with a 4-year history of progressive seventh nerve paresis progressing to total paralysis. Geniculate ganglion hemangioma and nerve resected en bloc. **(A)** Axial noncontrast computed tomography (CT) (left) and coronal noncontrast CT (right) demonstrate the hemangioma (*arrows*) enlarging the geniculate portion of the seventh nerve canal with extension into the proximal tympanic portion of the seventh nerve canal.

(B) Axial noncontrast T1-weighted magnetic resonance imaging (MRI) (left) and axial contrast-enhanced T1-weighted MRI (right) demonstrate the expected intense enhancement of the hemangioma (*arrows*). Note the absence of osseous invasion, making differentiation of this hemangioma from an equally common (for these imaging characteristics and this location) schwannoma impossible.

A *congenital cholesteatoma* has well-defined osseous margins, but most importantly, does not demonstrate enhancement on contrast-enhanced MRI.

Perineural spread by neoplasm tends to occur when carcinomas extend through the skull base and involves the more distal portions of the facial nerve canal, which are uncommon locations for hemangiomas. Often there is a history of previously treated parotid or skull base neoplasm.

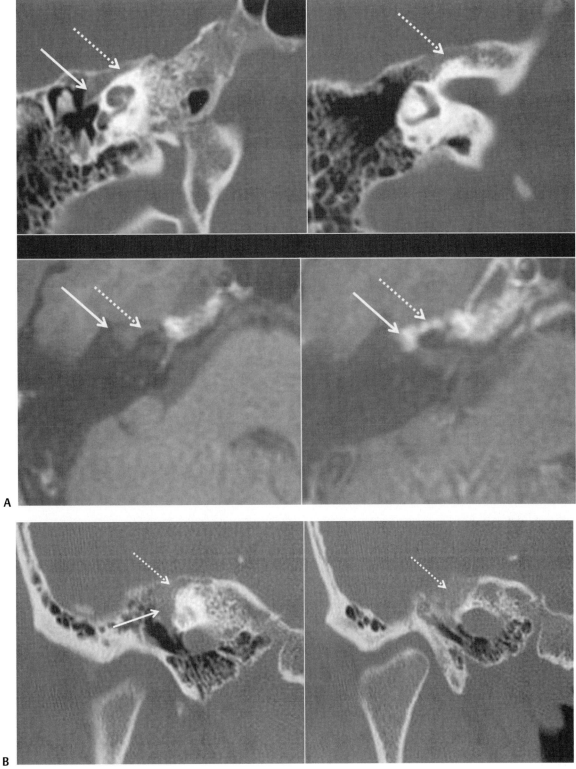

A

B

Figure 26–2 A 36-year-old man with a history of slowly progressive right facial paresis over several years. Surgery revealed hemangioma invading petrous temporal bone. **(A)** Contiguous axial noncontrast CT scans (top) and axial pre- and postcontrast T1-weighted MR scans (bottom) demonstrate the enhancing hemangioma centered in the geniculate ganglion region (*solid arrows*) with invasion of the contiguous petrous temporal bone (*dotted arrows*). **(B)** Coronal noncontrast CT scans (the left image is anterior to the right image) demonstrate the geniculate region hemangioma (*solid arrow*) and the anteromedial petrous tip osseous extension (*dotted arrows*) of the lesion. Note the intense enhancement of the hemangioma on the contrast-enhanced T1-weighted MRI scan. Also note the ill-defined margins and "honeycomb" appearance of the intraosseous portion of the lesion on the CT scan, which classifies this hemangioma as an ossifying hemangioma, helping to distinguish it from a schwannoma.

PEARLS _____

- The typical clinical story for a geniculate region hemangioma is an adult with a relatively short (e.g., several week) history of isolated progressive facial nerve palsy. One should evaluate the geniculate fossa region for an ill-defined mass (which enhances intensely on MRI) and demonstrates associated "honeycomb" osseous changes on a noncontrast CT.
- If the history includes sensorineural hearing loss and progressive seventh nerve palsy, an internal auditory canal region lesion should suspected. The workup should start with a contrast-enhanced MRI to search for areas of intense enhancement in the internal auditory canal (and geniculate fossa and posterior genu) regions. If negative, a temporal bone CT study to search for more subtle contour abnormalities along the course of the facial nerve canal should be considered.

Suggested Readings

Gebarski SS, Telian SA, Niparko JK. Enhancement along the normal facial nerve in the facial canal: MR imaging and anatomic correlation. Radiology 1992;183:391–394

Harnsberger HR, ed. Diagnostic Imaging: Head and Neck. Salt Lake City: Amirsys, 2004

Mangham CA, Carberry JN, Brackman DE. Management of intratemporal vascular tumors. Laryngoscope 1981;91:867–876

Piccirillo E, Agarwal M, Rohit MS, Khrais T, Sanna M. Management of temporal bone hemangiomas. Ann Otol Rhinol Laryngol 2004;113:431–437

Swartz JD, Harnsberger HR, eds. Imaging of the Temporal Bone, 3rd ed. New York: Thieme, 1998

Tokyol G, Yilmaz MD. Middle ear hemangioma: a case report. Am J Otolaryngol 2003;24:405–407

CHAPTER 27 Meningioma

Douglas J. Quint

Epidemiology

Meningiomas represent up to 18% of all intracranial tumors, with 7% of intracranial meningiomas arising on the anterior or posterior walls of the temporal bone.

Middle ear meningiomas are rare tumors that essentially always represent intratemporal extension of more common intracranial meningiomas. Like meningiomas in general, they are most often seen in middle-aged women. True primary middle ear meningiomas are very rare and remain reportable.

Clinical Features

Most patients present with posterior fossa symptoms due to the bulk of the meningioma arising at the skull base with the temporal bone involvement representing secondary extension. However, a chronic history of conductive hearing loss, tinnitus, otalgia, facial nerve palsy, or chronic otitis has been reported as a presenting symptom in patients with meningioma involving the temporal bone. This is not entirely surprising, as meningiomas are usually slow-growing tumors that can become quite large within the intracranial compartment while remaining clinically silent.

Pathology

Temporal bone meningiomas are histologically similar to typical intracranial meningiomas. They are considered benign lesions.

True primary middle ear meningiomas, if they exist, probably arise from ectopic neural crest arachnoidal cells.

Treatment

Aggressive surgery to remove the temporal bone portion of the lesion is the treatment of choice, particularly when middle ear symptoms are present. No chemotherapy is necessary, as these lesions are benign. Radiation therapy is reserved for recurrent, nonoperable lesions.

Imaging Findings

Most of these lesions are associated with a larger posterior fossa component with imaging characteristics typical of meningioma. However, the extremely rare, purely intratemporal meningioma appears as a nonspecific benign-appearing, nonaggressive mass.

CT

Thin-section (1 to 2 mm) noncontrast computed tomography (CT) performed in the axial and coronal planes and reconstructed with a detail (bone) algorithm best delineate the temporal bone and its contents. Sagittal reformatted images are also sometimes useful. Small middle ear meningiomas, and ossicular or temporal bone erosion or sclerotic/permeative changes due to frank intraosseous invasion by meningioma (due to intratemporal extension by a contiguous posterior fossa meningioma) are best delineated on CT scans.

No contrast-enhanced CT imaging is necessary to evaluate meningioma involvement of the temporal bone. However, if magnetic resonance imgaging (MRI) is not available, contrast-enhanced CT scans reconstructed at brain windows to search for an enhancing posterior fossa mass (e.g., the primary portion of the meningioma) contiguous with the temporal bone findings can be performed (**Fig. 27–1A**).

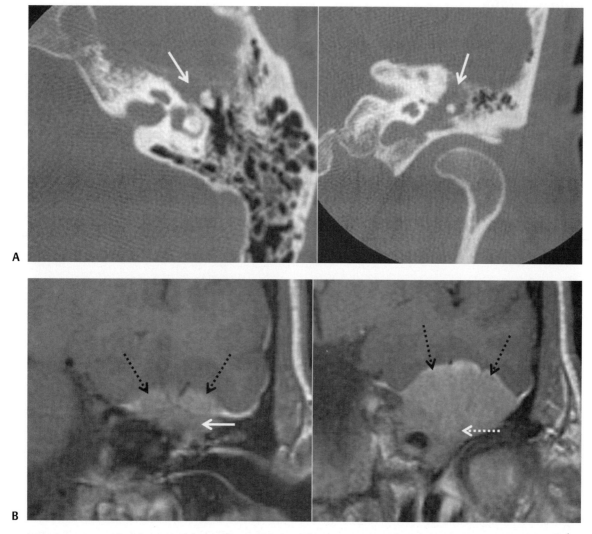

Figure 27–1 A 31-year-old man with a 4-month history of left ear fullness, decreased hearing, and occasional left ear "popping" sensations. A failed response to treatment for otitis media resulted in a computed tomography (CT) scan that revealed a large tumor that proved to be a meningioma at surgery. **(A)** Axial noncontrast CT (left) and coronal noncontrast CT (right) through the left temporal bone demonstrate abnormal soft tissue (*arrows*) invading and destroying por- tions of the tegmen tympani and anterior temporal bone wall with extension into the middle ear cleft to the region of the ossicles. **(B)** Coronal contrast-enhanced fat-suppressed T1-weighted MRI scans demonstrate the large meningioma contiguous with the temporal bone (*black dotted arrows*) frankly invading the temporal bone (*white arrows*), including the region of the middle ear (*white solid arrow*). *(Continued)*

MRI

The extent of intraosseous, intracranial (in particular meningeal in the case of meningiomas), and dural vascular involvement by neoplasm is best delineated on thin-section multiplanar fat-suppressed T2-weighted and noncontrast and contrast-enhanced T1-weighted MRI. Distinguishing trapped middle ear and mastoid secretions from tumor is also best achieved with MRI (**Fig. 27–1B,C**).

Like intracranial meningiomas, intratemporal meningiomas (or the intratemporal portion of primarily intracranial meningiomas) are usually isointense to brain on T1-weighted scans, homogeneously enhance in 90% of lesions on contrast-enhanced T1-weighted scans, and demonstrate signal either isointense or slightly hyperintense to brain on T2-weighted scans (**Fig. 27–1C**).

Angiography

If, after CT and MRI, a paraganglioma remains a differential diagnostic possibility, angiography can be performed preoperatively. Meningiomas demonstrate less vascularity than paragangliomas at angiography.

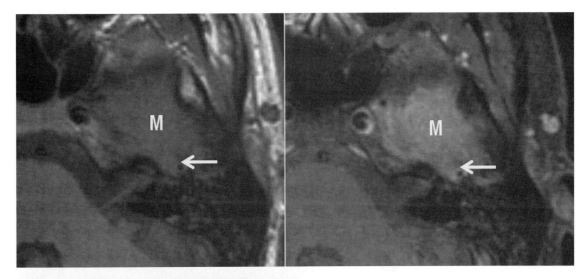

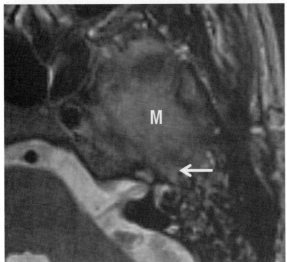

Figure 27–1 *(Continued)* **(C)** Axial pre- (left) and post-contrast (right) fat-suppressed T1-weighted MRI scans (top) and axial T2-weighted scan (bottom) demonstrate the large homogeneously enhancing predominantly intracranial meningioma (M) with a small portion of the tumor invading the middle ear cleft (*arrows*) as better delineated in **A.** As expected, the vast majority of temporal bone meningiomas represent intratemporal extension by an intracranial lesion contiguous with the temporal bone. The "typical" appearance is of a meningioma (signal similar to brain on T1- and T2- weighted scans with homogeneous enhancement). The clinical history reflects a lack of intracranial-related symptoms despite the large size of this lesion. It is difficult to delineate the middle ear involvement on the MRI relative to the CT study.

C

Differential Diagnosis

If the middle ear component of the lesion represents extension of an intracranial mass that has the typical benign appearance of a meningioma, then the differential diagnosis is limited, because the imaging appearance of meningiomas (and the differential diagnosis) is well known and quite limited.

If a lesion is localized to the temporal bone (in particular the middle ear region) without a definite intracranial component, the differential diagnosis includes other more common relatively non–aggressive-appearing intrinsic temporal bone (middle ear and mastoid) masses including schwannoma, paraganglioma, small nonaggressive adenomas and carcinoids, and even small primary or secondary malignancies.

PEARLS _____

- Diagnosis of a middle ear meningioma should prompt MRI evaluation of the posterior fossa to search for a primary lesion that has secondarily invaded the temporal bone.
- To this extent, one should be careful to use a large enough intracranial field of view when performing CT or MRI, as the intracranial components of meningiomas that have invaded the temporal bone can be extensive.

Suggested Readings

DeWeese DD, Everts EC. Primary intratympanic meningioma. Arch Otolaryngol 1972;96:62–66

El-Ghazali TMS. Primary intratympanic meningioma. J Laryngol Otol 1981;95:849–852

Ferlito A, Devaney KO, Rinaldo A. Primary extracranial meningioma in the vicinity of the temporal bone: a benign lesion which is rarely recognized clinically. Acta Otolaryngol 2004;124:5–7

Harnsberger HR, ed. Diagnostic Imaging: Head and Neck. Salt Lake City: Amirsys, 2004

Lawand A, Walker AN, Griffin J. Pathology quiz case. Middle ear meningioma. Arch Otolaryngol Head Neck Surg 2002;128:975–977

Prayson RA. Middle ear meningiomas. Ann Diagn Pathol 2000;4:149–153

Rietz DR, Ford CN, Kurtycz DF, Brandenburg JH, Hafez GR. Significance of apparent intratympanic meningiomas. Laryngoscope 1983;93:1397–1404

Rojas R, Palacios E, D'Antonio M. An unusual primary intratympanic meningioma. Ear Nose Throat J 2004;83:607–608

CHAPTER 28 Squamous Cell Carcinoma (Middle Ear)
Douglas J. Quint

Epidemiology

Primary middle ear squamous cell carcinoma is a rare neoplasm seen in less than 1 in 10,000 patients presenting with otologic disease. It is less common than primary external auditory canal squamous cell carcinoma.

This rare carcinoma is most often seen in 50- to 60-year-old men. It is associated with chronic otitis media, which is associated with increased cellular metaplasia due to ongoing inflammation/otorrhea possibly mediated through human papilloma virus (which is present in many of these patients). These carcinomas are also associated with prior radiation therapy.

These patients have a poor prognosis, as most present with advanced disease (e.g., temporal bone or intracranial extension) and it is difficult, if not impossible, to achieve complete neoplasm resection because many crucial structures are nearby (brain, skull base internal carotid artery, cavernous sinus, dural venous sinuses, etc.). Five-year survival is less than 50% in patients who are treated with surgery and radiation therapy.

Clinical Features

These patients present with a long history of ear symptoms, namely pain, discharge, bleeding, and refractory granulation formation. These patients may also have facial palsy reflecting involvement of the tympanic portion of cranial nerve VII. Sudden deafness can be seen late in the course of the disease. The clinical scenario of seventh nerve palsy, deafness, and continuing otorrhea should suggest a middle ear process. The diagnosis is often initially overlooked, as middle ear squamous cell carcinoma is a rare entity and all of the symptoms seen in these patients (except for the facial nerve palsy) are typical of chronic otitis media.

Pathology

Middle ear squamous cell carcinoma probably arises from tympanic mucosa. Temporal bone squamous cell carcinomas are considered stage 1 and 2 when limited to the external auditory canal. By definition, they are considered stage 3 when they involve the middle ear (stage 4 lesions involve the temporal bone more extensively). Cases of primary middle ear squamous cell carcinoma are so rare that there are no reliable statistics as to whether these lesions metastasize. As mentioned above, these patients have a poor prognosis primarily due to their overall late presentation.

Treatment

Treatment for middle ear (and all temporal bone) squamous cell carcinomas includes surgery, chemotherapy, and postsurgical radiation therapy. In cases of extensive disease, palliative radiation therapy only may be performed.

Imaging Findings

As most of these lesions present at a relatively late stage, frank invasion and destruction of portions of the temporal bone is often already present. The extent of temporal bone (including ossicular) destruction is best assessed with computed tomography (CT), whereas delineating trapped secretions from invasive tumor and defining the extent of extratemporal involvement (intracranial, intravascular, infratemporal, etc.) is best assessed with magnetic resonance imaging (MRI).

Soft tissue masses in the middle ear cleft are usually nonspecific in appearance on CT and MRI, consistent with both inflammatory and neoplastic processes.

CT

High-resolution (1–2 mm) noncontrast CT performed in the axial and coronal planes and reconstructed with a "detail" (bone) algorithm best delineates the extent of temporal bone (including ossicular) involvement. Occasionally, sagittal reformatted images may prove valuable. If MRI is not available, intracranial, infratemporal, and vascular involvement can be grossly assessed by contrast-enhanced CT, but usually the extent of disease is best assessed with MRI and no contrast-enhanced CT imaging is necessary (**Fig. 28–1**). Contrast-enhanced CT can be used to search for associated cervical adenopathy.

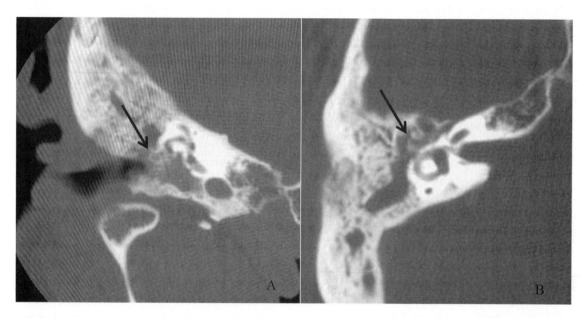

Figure 28–1 A 44-year-old man presents with a 2-year history of right ear itching, with minimal associated pain and drainage. Biopsy revealed squamous cell carcinoma. Coronal (left) and axial (right) noncontrast computed tomography (CT) scans through the right temporal bone demonstrate abnormal right external and middle ear region soft tissue (*arrows*) with associated temporal bone and ossicular destruction. It is impossible to differentiate trapped secretions from tumor. After failing to tolerate radiation therapy, surgery confirmed the unresectable nature of the tumor, which involved the entire middle ear including the geniculate, tympanic, and the second genu portions of the seventh nerve and the region of the carotid artery and eustachian tube.

MRI

Thin-section multiplanar pre- and postcontrast T1- and T2-weighted scanning is best for delineating the extent of intrinsic and extrinsic temporal bone carcinoma **(Fig. 28–2)**. The extent of intraosseous, intracranial, vascular, and extracranial (subtemporal, scalp, external ear) spread by neoplasm, and perineural spread by neoplasm is best delineated on multiplanar fat-suppressed T2 and contrast-enhanced T1 MRI. Distinguishing trapped middle ear and mastoid secretions from tumor is also best achieved with MRI. Cervical lymph nodes can also be detected on fat-suppressed contrast-enhanced MRI for staging purposes.

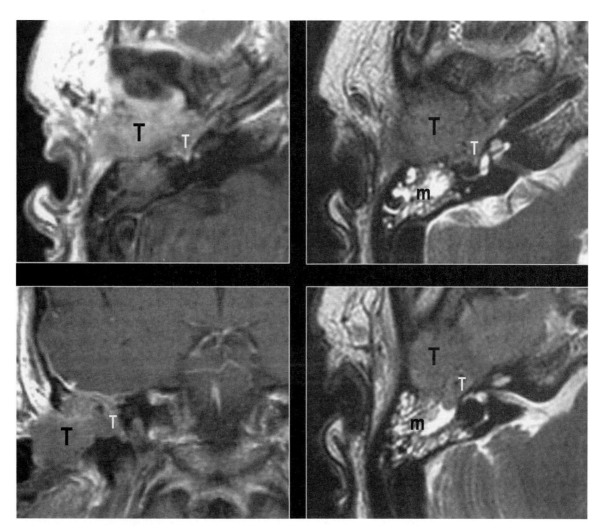

Figure 28–2 A 56-year-old woman presents with 6 months of right oral "fullness," several weeks of hemorrhagic otorrhea, and 2 days of right-sided facial paresis. Imaging revealed a temporal bone mass that at biopsy proved to be squamous cell carcinoma. Axial (upper left) and coronal (lower left) contrast-enhanced T1-weighted and axial T2-weighted (upper and lower right) magnetic resonance imaging (MRI) scans through the right temporal bone region demonstrates the enhancing right temporal bone carcinoma (*black T*) centered in the external auditory canal region with temporomandibular joint region and middle ear region (*white T*) extension. The T2-weighted MRI scans permit differentiation of tumor (isointense to brain) from mastoid-trapped secretions (m), which is difficult on the contrast-enhanced T1-weighted scans and is impossible on CT scans.

Differential Diagnosis

Imaging findings are nonspecific. Other more common middle ear inflammatory or aggressive neoplastic processes should always be considered in these patients.

Symptoms of an aggressive or *chronic otitis media* can mimic middle ear squamous cell carcinoma and are much more common clinical entities than carcinoma. An aggressive *jugulotympanic paraganglioma* can present similar to a temporal bone carcinoma, but is a more common neoplastic process. Other malignancies that are more commonly seen than primary middle ear carcinoma include metastatic disease, malignant adenomatous tumors, sarcomas (particularly in children), and perineural spread by adenoid cystic carcinoma or extratemporal squamous cell carcinoma.

PEARLS _____

- In the setting of chronic, recurrent inflammatory disease of the middle ear, new facial paralysis or acute hearing loss should prompt a search for carcinoma with aggressive CT imaging.
- Once a destructive, permeative temporal bone process has been detected with CT scanning, the extent of disease with special attention to intracranial, vascular, and subtemporal involvement is best delineated with MRI.
- Cervical adenopathy can be assessed with either CT or MRI. Detecting extratemporal involvement by this carcinoma affects management.

Suggested Readings

Agada FO, Gnananandha C, Wickham M. Squamous cell carcinoma of the middle ear: case report and literature review. Annals of African Medicine 2004;3:90–92

Suzuki K, Takahashi M, Ito Y, et al. Bilateral middle ear squamous cell carcinoma and clinical review of an additional 5 cases of middle ear carcinomas. Auris Nasus Larynx 1999;26:33–38

Swartz JD, Harnsberger HR, eds. Imaging of the Temporal Bone, 3rd ed. New York: Thieme, 1998

Takano A, Takasaki K, Kumagami H, Higami Y, Kobayashi T. Clinical records: a case of bilateral middle-ear squamous cell carcinoma. J Laryngol Otol 2001;115:815–818

CHAPTER 29 Adenomatous Lesion

Douglas J. Quint

Epidemiology

The neoplasms discussed in this chapter (middle ear adenomas, carcinoids, adenocarcinoma, and endolymphatic sac tumors) are considered different types of adenomatous lesions and are each very rare.

Clinical Features

Middle ear adenomas and carcinoids are nonaggressive neoplasms that can present clinically in a manner similar to other more common benign middle ear masses such as primary or secondary cholesteatoma or paraganglioma. They appear as a retrotympanic mass at otoscopy. Symptoms include a feeling of ear "fullness," tinnitus, and conductive hearing loss. These lesions usually do not involve the facial nerve and therefore do not present with seventh nerve palsy.

Middle ear endolymphatic sac tumors are more aggressive neoplasms and often present with seventh nerve involvement in addition to the above-described symptoms.

Adenocarcinomas of the middle ear, being an aggressive process, present in a manner similar to other aggressive middle ear processes. Specifically, such lesions present with otorrhea, otalgia, and facial nerve paralysis. These patients often have a long clinical otologic history (e.g., chronic otitis media).

Pathology

Adenomatous (glandular) lesions of the middle ear region include several different entities, all of which are probably histologically related. These include middle ear adenomas, carcinoids, adenocarcinomas, and endolymphatic sac tumors.

Middle ear adenomas and carcinoids most likely represent the same entity classically believed to arise from epithelial tissues of the middle ear. Recent work suggests that they may arise from nondifferentiated endodermal stem cells. They are hypovascular lesions demonstrating a nonaggressive, nonpapillary, or pleomorphic histologic pattern with varying amounts of glandular and endocrine differentiation (e.g., carcinoids have more neuroendocrine differentiation than adenomas).

True adenocarcinomas of the temporal bone may arise from the mucosal lining of the middle ear or nondifferentiated endodermal stem cells. Histologically, they have an aggressive, usually nonpapillary appearance. They can invade ossicles or nearby bone and the intracranial compartment.

Endolymphatic duct tumors (also called aggressive papillary adenocarcinomas of the temporal bone) can be seen in the middle ear, though they probably arise in the endolymphatic sac or duct. They are vascular lesions and demonstrate an aggressive papillary histologic pattern.

Treatment

Adenomas and carcinoids are treated surgically. Complete resection is curative. Nonpapillary and papillary (endolymphatic sac tumors) adenocarcinomas have usually spread within the temporal bone or extended locally outside the temporal bone at the time of presentation. Radical surgery followed by radiation therapy is usually performed. The aggressive papillary tumors of the temporal bone (endo-

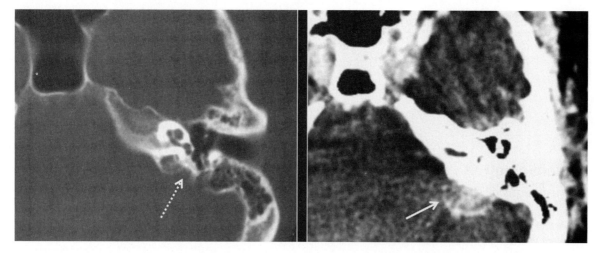

Figure 29–1 A 49-year-old man with hearing loss. Endolymphatic sac tumor (papillary adenocarcinoma); partially resected. Axial contrast-enhanced computed tomography (CT) sections through the left temporal bone [bone windows (right); and soft tissue windows (left)], demonstrate enlargement of the vestibular aqueduct region (*dotted arrow*) by the tumor that also extends into the posterior cranial fossa (*solid arrow*) in the region of the endolymphatic sac.

lymphatic sac tumors) respond well to resection. Nonpapillary ("true") adenocarcinomas have a poor prognosis.

Imaging Findings

CT

Thin-section (1 to 2 mm) noncontrast computed tomography (CT) performed in the axial and coronal planes and reconstructed with a "detail" (bone) algorithm best delineate the temporal bone and its contents. Sagittal reformatted images are also sometimes useful. In patients with these lesions, middle ear masses and temporal bone destruction is best delineated on CT scans. Contrast-enhanced CT scans are not useful for evaluation of these lesions (**Fig. 29–1**).

MRI

The extent of intraosseous, intracranial, vascular, and extracranial spread by neoplasm, and perineural spread by neoplasm is best delineated on thin-section multiplanar fat-suppressed T2 and noncontrast and contrast-enhanced T1-weighted magnetic resonance imaging (MRI). Distinguishing trapped middle ear and mastoid secretions from tumor is also best achieved with MRI.

Middle ear adenomas and carcinoids present as nonaggressive middle ear masses without osseous destruction, associated chronic otitis media, or mastoid inflammatory changes. They often encase the ossicles. Only multiplanar noncontrast CT scans are necessary to define the extent of these middle ear lesions. No contrast-enhanced CT scans are necessary. These lesions are relatively nonspecific in appearance on MRI, demonstrating decreased signal on T1-weighted scans, mixed signal on T2-weighted scans, and modest contrast enhancement (**Fig. 29–2**).

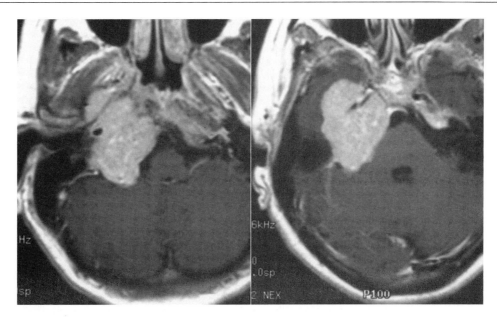

Figure 29–2 A 42-year-old woman with right-sided tinnitus and facial numbness with hoarseness, ataxia, and right-eye diplopia. Limited surgery revealed adenocarcinoma. Axial contrast-enhanced T1-weighted scans through the right temporal bone demonstrate a large enhancing mass involving the right middle ear cleft and petrous tip regions with additional middle cranial fossa, cavernous sinus and posterior fossa extension. As described in the text, these lesions tend to be large at presentation often with extratemporal spread. This patient was treated with limited resection and extensive radiation and continues to do well 12 years later.

Adenocarcinomas are more aggressive lesions that have often already invaded the temporal bone or destroyed ossicles by the time they present. These lesions can extend intracranially, below the skull base or into the external auditory canal or scalp regions. Although osseous involvement is best delineated on noncontrast CT scanning, the extent of temporal and extratemporal spread of neoplasm is best assessed with MRI. The MRI characteristics are similar to those of adenomas and are again not specific. It is the extent of disease that suggests a more aggressive neoplastic process.

Angiography

If paraganglioma remains a differential diagnostic possibility based on the location of the lesion on CT and MRI, then formal endovascular angiography could be performed preoperatively.

Differential Diagnosis

As each of these lesions is very rare, more common processes should first be ruled out. Before considering the diagnosis of a middle ear adenoma or carcinoid, much more common primary or secondary cholesteatomas should be considered. Depending on the location of a middle ear lesion, a glomus tympanicum paraganglioma may also be in the differential diagnosis.

Other lesions with imaging appearances similar if not identical to that seen with adenocarcinomas include aggressive inflammatory processes or jugulotympanicum tumors, metastatic disease, or a rare squamous cell carcinoma.

PEARL

- Due to the rarity of these lesions and their lack of specific associated clinical symptoms and imaging features, other more common lesions should always be considered first in a differential diagnosis. One must rule out metastases (metastatic adenocarcinoma) before diagnosing a primary adenocarcinoma of the temporal bone).

Suggested Readings

Dadas B, Alkan S, Turgut S, Basak T. Primary papillary adenocarcinoma confined to the middle ear and mastoid. Eur Arch Otorhinolaryngol 2001;258:93–95

Harnsberger HR, ed. Diagnostic Imaging: Head and Neck. Salt Lake City: Amirsys, 2004

Maintz D, Stupp C, Krueger K, Wustrow J, Lackner K. MRI and CT of adenomatous tumors of the middle ear. Neuroradiology 2001;43:58–61

Paulus W, Romstock J, Weidenbecher M, Huk WJ, Fahlbusch R. Middle ear adenocarcinoma with intracranial extension. J Neurosurg 1999;90:555–558

Swartz JD, Harnsberger HR, eds. Imaging of the Temporal Bone, 3rd ed. New York: Thieme, 1998

Torske KR, Thompson LDR. Adenoma versus carcinoid tumor of the middle ear: a study of 48 cases and review of the literature. Mod Pathol 2002;15:543–555

CHAPTER 30 Adenoid Cystic Carcinoma
Douglas J. Quint

Epidemiology

Twenty-five percent of all salivary gland tumors arise from minor salivary glands, and 50% of minor salivary gland tumors are malignant. The smaller the minor salivary gland, the greater the risk that a tumor arising from that gland is malignant. The most common primary minor salivary gland malignancy is adenoid cystic carcinoma. As salivary gland tissue is rarely found in the middle ear (choristomas), it is possible that occasional primary minor salivary gland malignancies will occur in the middle ear. Less than a dozen such primary cases have been reported. Most adenoid cystic carcinomas of the middle ear region secondarily involve the middle ear as a result of cephalad perineural spread of a parotid gland adenoid cystic carcinoma along the seventh cranial nerve into the temporal bone.

Clinical Features

Primary middle ear adenoid cystic carcinoma is so rare that no specific clinical features can be described. As it is considered an aggressive tumor that can invade osseous structures (in this case, the temporal bone), it can be expected to present with pain, seventh nerve dysfunction, and conductive hearing loss depending on its extent. With invasion of the skull base or the intracranial compartment, additional cranial nerve and other symptoms may be present.

Perineural spread by adenoid cystic carcinoma along the facial nerve is often asymptomatic. However, it can present with progressive seventh nerve symptoms and possibly hearing loss depending on the extent of middle ear involvement. An otherwise asymptomatic parotid mass may be palpable.

Pathology

Primary temporal bone adenoid cystic carcinomas are considered a type of malignant ceruminous gland tumor (along with ceruminous adenocarcinomas) that usually arise in the external auditory canal as there is normally no salivary gland tissue in the middle ear. These are very rare tumors in the middle ear region. When they arise in the middle ear region, they are believed to arise from either ectopic salivary gland tissue (which has been identified in the middle ear region in pathologic studies) or multipotential middle ear mucosal cells (endodermal stem cells).

Treatment

Therapy involves surgery, radiation therapy, or chemotherapy depending on the extent of disease.

Imaging Findings

Primary middle ear adenoid cystic carcinoma is indistinguishable from other aggressive middle ear neoplasms (e.g., squamous cell carcinoma, malignant adenomatous tumors, sarcomas) and some aggressive infections. Defining the extent of disease determines if surgery is a therapeutic option.

CT

High-resolution (1 to 2 mm) computed tomography (CT) scanning performed in the axial and coronal planes and reconstructed with a "detail" (bone) algorithm best evaluates the temporal bone region for small soft tissue lesions in the middle ear cleft, facial nerve canal enlargement, and frank osseous destruction. Occasionally, sagittal reformatted images may also prove valuable. If magnetic resonance imaging (MRI) is not available, intracranial, infratemporal, and vascular involvement can be grossly assessed by contrast-enhanced CT, but usually such extent of disease is best assessed with MRI and no contrast-enhanced CT imaging is necessary.

MRI

The extent of intraosseous, vascular, intracranial, and extracranial spread by neoplasm, in addition to perineural spread by neoplasm, is best evaluated on multiplanar fat-suppressed T2-weighted and noncontrast and contrast-enhanced T1-weighted MRI. Distinguishing trapped secretions from tumor is also best achieved with MRI. Evaluation of the parotid gland in cases of suspected perineural spread of malignancy is also best done with MRI (**Fig. 30–1**).

Angiography

If paraganglioma remains a differential diagnostic possibility based on the location of the lesion on CT and MRI, then formal endovascular angiography could be performed preoperatively.

Differential Diagnosis

Imaging features of these very rare tumors are nonspecific. Other primary and secondary processes should be considered first in a differential diagnosis. The ultimate diagnosis can only be made pathologically.

Specifically, before considering a primary middle ear adenoid cystic carcinoma, other aggressive neoplastic (e.g., squamous cell carcinoma, malignant adenomatous tumors, sarcomas, metastatic disease, invasive jugulotympanic paraganglioma) or inflammatory (e.g., chronic otitis) processes should be considered.

When considering a secondary middle ear adenoid cystic carcinoma (e.g., perineural spread from an extratemporal source), other primary temporal bone tumors that can be found along the intratemporal seventh cranial nerve (e.g., schwannoma, hemangioma) and other neoplasms that can extend perineurally (e.g., squamous cell carcinoma, mucoepidermoid) need to be considered as do inflammatory/infectious processes (e.g., idiopathic Bell palsy, herpes zoster) that can affect the facial nerve.

PEARLS _____

- There are no specific clinical or imaging findings to suggest the rare diagnosis of primary middle ear adenoid cystic carcinoma.
- Other middle ear neoplasms (e.g., schwannoma, hemangioma) and infectious processes are much more common than adenoid cystic carcinomas of the temporal bone. In patients with known or previously treated parotid malignancy, perineural extension by neoplasm should always be considered.
- Enlargement of the facial canal by perineural spread of neoplasm may not be accompanied by seventh nerve symptoms if the nerve has not yet been invaded by neoplasm.
- Enhancement of the intratemporal seventh nerve without enlargement of the facial nerve canal can represent infiltration by tumor.

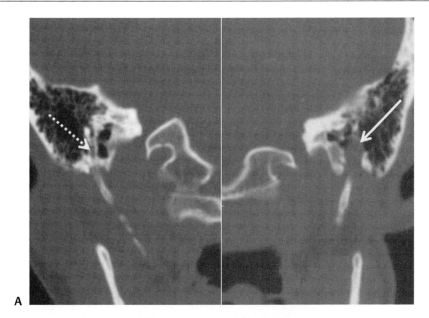

A

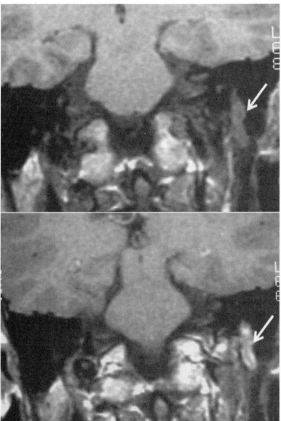

B

Figure 30–1 A 48-year-old with recurrent adenoid cystic carcinoma extending cephalad from the parotid surgical site into and enlarging the descending portion of the left facial canal. **(A)** A normal descending facial nerve canal on the right (*dotted arrow*) and an enlarged descending facial nerve canal on the left (*solid arrow*). **(B)** Noncontrast T1-weighted MRI (top); contrast T1-weighted MRI (bottom) demonstrates the enhancing neoplasm (*arrows*) within the left descending facial nerve canal.

- Enhancement of the intratemporal portion of the seventh nerve without associated seventh nerve enlargement can represent neoplasm or infection. Follow-up imaging in 3 to 4 months in these patients to assess for interval resolution of the enhancement (which essentially rules out tumor) is suggested before diagnosing a neoplasm.

Suggested Readings

Cannon CR, McLean WC. Adenoid cystic carcinoma of the middle ear and temporal bone. Otolaryngol Head Neck Surg 1983;91:96–99

Harnsberger HR, ed. Diagnostic Imaging: Head and Neck. Salt Lake City: Amirsys, 2004

Morrow TA, Baredes S, Jahn AF, Schulder M. Pathologic quiz case 2. Adenoid cystic carcinoma. Arch Otolaryngol Head Neck Surg 1991;117:804–805, 807–808

Som PM, Curtin HD, eds. Head and Neck Imaging, 4th ed. St. Louis: Mosby, 2003

Swartz JD, Harnsberger HR, eds. Imaging of the Temporal Bone, 3rd ed. New York: Thieme, 1998

Douglas J. Quint

Epidemiology

Rhabdomyosarcoma is the second most common pediatric head and neck malignancy and the most common soft tissue sarcoma in children. Rhabdomyosarcomas constitute 3% of all malignancies in patients younger than 20 years old.

Rhabdomyosarcomas are the most common primary temporal bone malignancy in children. These tumors most commonly present in children younger than 5 years old or in their late teens.

Approximately 7 to 8% of head and neck rhabdomyosarcomas involve the middle ear or mastoid regions (the nasopharynx and orbit are more common locations for these tumors).

In the middle ear and mastoid regions, these tumors are usually invasive and, as they are located near meninges, tend to spread intracranially. They are often unresectable at the time of diagnosis and have a relatively poorer prognosis than other head and neck rhabdomyosarcomas. However, less than 30% of patients have local metastases at presentation and there is an 85 to 90% three-year survival in these patients.

Clinical Features

Presenting symptoms are similar to those of chronic otitis media (which is a much more common diagnosis particularly in children), which is why the correct diagnosis is often delayed. Symptoms are similar to other middle ear processes including hearing loss, ear pain, ear discharge, and sometimes a bleeding external auditory canal (EAC) polyp. Facial nerve paralysis is unusual. The presence of an EAC polyp in a patient with chronic otitis should suggest the possibility of an underlying neoplasm.

Pathology

Rhabdomyosarcomas are highly malignant mesenchymal (skeletal muscle origin) tumors that are usually unresectable at presentation. There are three histologic types: embryonal (>75% of tumors), alveolar, and pleomorphic.

Treatment

Most tumors are not totally resectable at the time of diagnosis. Treatment usually entails debulking surgery (at which time the diagnosis is made) followed by multiagent chemotherapy and radiation therapy. Improvements in chemotherapeutic and radiation treatment protocols have resulted in up to 90% three-year survival in recent studies.

Imaging Findings

Like most malignancies of the temporal bone (and particularly the middle ear region), imaging is nonspecific and is performed to assess the extent of disease. Rhabdomyosarcomas of the temporal bone tend to be unresectable at presentation, so it is particularly important to define the extent of (extratemporal) spread of neoplasm before initiating therapy.

CT

Thin-section (1 to 2 mm) noncontrast computed tomography (CT) performed in the axial and coronal planes and reconstructed with a "detail" (bone) algorithm best delineates the temporal bone and its contents. Sagittal reformatted images are also sometimes useful. In patients with rhabdomyosarcomas, middle ear involvement and ossicular and temporal bone invasion with frank osseous destruction are best delineated on CT scans. Contrast-enhanced CT scans are not useful for evaluation of these lesions (**Fig. 31–1**).

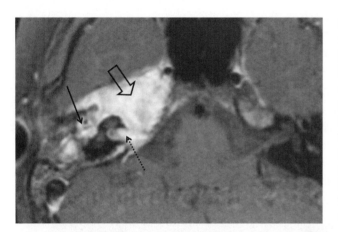

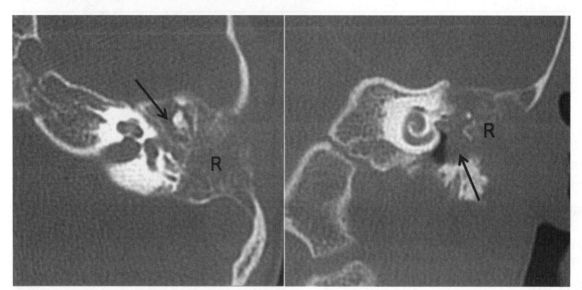

Figure 31–1 10-year-old girl with a 1 month history of intermittent right-sided headaches and dizziness upon standing and a several-week history of a progressive right facial droop. Axial contrast-enhanced fat-suppressed T1-weighted magnetic resonance (MR) imaging demonstrates a large mass replacing much of the tympanic and petrous portions of the temporal bone (*large arrow*) with middle ear (*solid arrow*) and internal auditory canal (*dotted arrow*) involvement. Mastoidectomy with biopsy revealed embryonal rhabdomyosarcoma. (*Note*: As with many aggressive temporal bone tumors, this patient presented when the mass was large and unresectable.) *Note*: While impossible to rule out vascular (sigmoid sinus) invasion on the CT scan, the normal flow void on the MR imaging essentially rules out such vascular invasion.

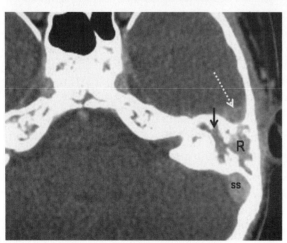

Figure 31–2(A) A 7-year-old boy with a 1-week history of left ear bloody otorrhea and slight left-sided hearing loss. He was treated for possible otitis externa, but at a 1-week follow-up clinic visit, a residual external auditory canal mass was seen; biopsy revealed embryonal rhabdomyosarcoma. Axial contrast-enhanced left temporal bone region computed tomography (CT) scan (bone window images above; brain window image below left; coronal bone window, upper right) demonstrates a soft tissue mass destroying the mastoid portion of the left temporal bone (R) with middle ear involvement (*black arrows*). Intracranial extension is seen extending into the middle cranial fossa (*dotted white arrow*). Similar enhancement is seen in the region of the left sigmoid sinus (ss); this latter enhancement is consistent with normal vascular enhancement or spread of neoplasm. (*Continued*)

A

MRI

The extent of intraosseous, intracranial (in particular meningeal), vascular, extracranial (subtemporal), and perineural spread by neoplasm is best delineated on thin-section multiplanar fat-suppressed T2-weighted and noncontrast and contrast-enhanced T1-weighted magnetic resonance imaging (MRI). Distinguishing trapped middle ear and mastoid secretions from tumor is also best achieved with MRI.

Magnetic resonance imaging characteristics of these lesions are nonspecific, including low to intermediate signal on T1-weighted scans, variable signal on T2-weighted scans, and enhancement on contrast-enhanced T1-weighted scans (**Fig. 31–2**).

Less than 30% of temporal bone rhabdomyosarcomas have local metastases at the time of presentation. Although CT and MRI can demonstrate morphologically abnormal lymph nodes that might suggest spread of neoplasm, metabolic fluorodeoxyglucose positron emission tomography (FDG-PET) evaluation can identify malignant nodes before they demonstrate pathologic morphology.

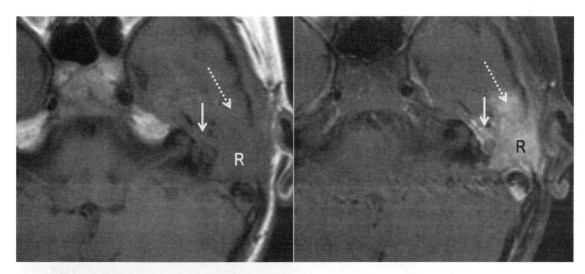

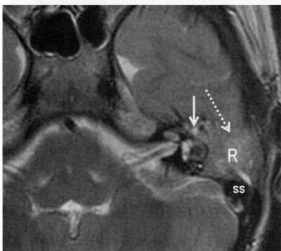

Figure 31–2 *(Continued)* **(B)** Axial precontrast (upper left) and fat-suppressed contrast-enhanced (upper right) T1-weighted and axial T2-weighted (below) MRI scans through the left temporal bone demonstrates the extensive left temporal bone rhabdomyosarcoma (R), middle ear extension (*solid arrows*), and middle cranial fossa extension (*dotted arrows*). A normal flow void is seen in the region of the sigmoid sinus (ss). *Note:* As with many temporal bone tumors, this patient presented when the mass was large and unresectable. Also, the mass demonstrates signal isointense to the brain on the T2-weighted scans inconsistent with the trapped secretions. Finally, while impossible to rule out vascular (sigmoid sinus) invasion on the CT scan, the normal "flow void" on the MRI essentially rules out such vascular invasion.

B

Differential Diagnosis

Imaging features of these tumors are nonspecific. Other primary and secondary processes should also be considered in a differential diagnosis. The ultimate diagnosis can be made only at biopsy.

Other aggressive though less common temporal bone tumors such as squamous cell carcinoma, adenomatous tumors (adenocarcinoma, endolymphatic sac tumors, adenomas), and metastases should be considered, but are usually ruled out based on the age of the patient. Rhabdomyosarcoma may mimic chronic inflammation, but chronic otitis is far more common, particularly in children, and usually responds to medical therapy.

Langerhans histiocytosis can be difficult to differentiate from a temporal bone sarcoma in a child. Involvement of other bones is more consistent with histiocytosis, though biopsy may be necessary.

PEARLS

- As even extensive temporal bone rhabdomyosarcomas have been shown to be responsive to aggressive therapy, such a sarcoma should be considered in the differential diagnosis of any aggressive destructive temporal bone process in a child. In particular, in a child with an external auditory canal polyp and chronic otitis unresponsive to medical therapy, an underlying neoplasm should be considered.
- Complete evaluation of these lesions includes multiplanar CT and MRI and sometimes metabolic PET imaging to completely assess the extent of disease.

Suggested Readings

Harnsberger HR, ed. Diagnostic Imaging: Head and Neck. Salt Lake City: Amirsys, 2004

Hawkins DS, Anderson JR, Paides CN, et al. Improved outcome for patients with middle ear rhabdomyosarcoma: a children's oncology group study. J Clin Oncol 2001;19:3073–3079

Hu J, Liu S, Qiu J. Embryonal rhabdomyosarcoma of the middle ear. Otolaryngol Head Neck Surg 2002;126:690–692

Maroldi R, Farina D, Palvarini L, et al. Computed tomography and magnetic resonance imaging of pathologic conditions of the middle ear. Eur J Radiol 2001;40:78–93

Som PM, Curtin HD, eds. Head and Neck Imaging, 4th ed. St. Louis: Mosby, 2003

Swartz JD, Harnsberger HR, eds. Imaging of the Temporal Bone, 3rd ed. New York: Thieme, 1998

CHAPTER 32 Metastasis
Hemant Parmar

Epidemiology

Metastatic carcinoma of the middle ear is uncommon and rarely described in the literature. Metastatic middle ear tumors most often arise from breast, lung, kidney, prostate, stomach, thyroid, and esophagus, in descending order of frequency. In the head and neck region there are some reports of secondary middle ear tumors occurring as a result of direct extension of tumors such as nasopharyngeal carcinoma, salivary gland carcinoma, and maxillary tumors. In general, four routes of tumor metastasis from the primary sites to the temporal bone and middle ear can be considered: (1) blood-borne dissemination from a distant primary site, (2) direct invasion from an adjacent site, (3) diffuse metastatic leptomeningeal carcinomatosis, and (4) perineural spread.

Clinical Features

Generally, the clinical presentation depends on the extent of bone destruction. Patients present with complaints of ear pain, conductive deafness, tinnitus, and otorrhea. Bleeding from the ear and progressive facial paralysis are also reported. Aggressive lesions with intracranial extension and sigmoid sinus extension show symptoms of raised intracranial pressure, such as headache, vomiting, and bilateral blurry vision. Middle ear metastasis can present years after the treatment and cure of primary tumor.

Pathology

The majority of the middle ear metastases involve the bone. Facial nerve involvement is usually secondary. The intracanalicular portion of the facial nerve is most commonly involved, followed by the mastoid, tympanic, and labyrinthine segments. The facial nerve can be an important pathway of metastatic spread, and salivary gland tumors may spread retrograde along the nerve and extend into the middle ear. Extensive involvement of the temporal bone from the petrous apex to mastoid tip is also described. Histopathology of middle ear metastasis shows malignant cells, depending on the primary site of malignancy.

Treatment

Treatment for metastatic middle ear tumors is usually palliative. Combined surgical and chemotherapeutic treatment can be considered in some cases, based on the primary site of cancer. Intracranial complications need symptomatic treatment.

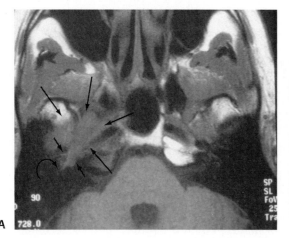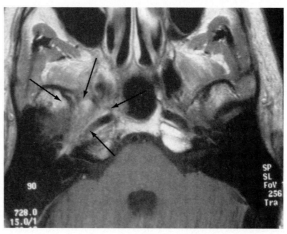

Figure 32–1 Metastatic adenoid cystic carcinoma. Axial T1-weighted images obtained **(A)** before and **(B)** after the use of intravenous contrast demonstrates an aggressive infiltrative mass involving the petrous apex (*straight large arrows*) and extending along the expected course of the greater superficial petrosal nerve (*small arrows*) and continuing along the tympanic segment of the facial nerve (*curved arrow*). **(B)** The lesion homogeneously enhances with contrast (*arrows*). This tumor originated in the parotid gland and represents perineural extension along the facial nerve extending into the middle ear cavity.

Imaging Findings

CT

Computed tomography (CT) scan appearances for middle ear metastasis are nonspecific and resemble those of other aggressive lesions of the middle ear. Tissue biopsy is required for diagnosis. Middle ear metastasis usually presents with a destructive soft tissue mass infiltrating the middle ear cavity and mastoid air cells. A varying degree of ossicular destruction is noted. Cases with involvement of the facial nerve demonstrate destruction of the facial nerve canal, especially at its anterior genu and the tympanic segment. There may even be widening at the level of the porus acusticus. A CT scan may be required to evaluate the bony skull base for additional lesions (**Fig. 32–1**).

MRI

Magnetic resonance imaging (MRI) is more sensitive than CT scan for soft tissue differentiation. Contrast-enhanced MRI is especially superior to CT in delineating a mass lesion along the facial nerve and demonstrates thickening and enhancement along the course of the facial nerve.

Magnetic resonance imaging is also better than CT for assessing metastasis involving the meninges, cerebral and cerebellar parenchyma, and brainstem.

IMAGING PEARLS _____

- Middle ear metastatic tumors are rare.
- Middle ear symptoms such as pain, conductive deafness, and bleeding in the presence of malignancy should raise suspicion of a middle ear metastasis.
- The presence of a second lesion in the base of the skull or elsewhere in the calvarium helps in establishing the diagnosis.
- CT scan shows an aggressive soft tissue lesion with permeative bone destruction.
- MRI is more sensitive than CT scan for soft tissue differentiation, especially along the facial nerve and for intracranial extent.

Suggested Readings

Hill BA, Kohut RA. Metastatic adenocarcinoma of the temporal bone. Arch Otolaryngol Head Neck Surg 1976;102:568–571

Imauchi Y, Kaga K, Nibu K, Sakuma N, Iino Y, Kodera K. Metastasis of cervical esophagus carcinoma to the temporal bone-a study of the temporal bone histology. Auris Nasus Larynx 2001;28:169–172

Nelson EG, Hinojosa R. Histopathology of metastatic temporal bone tumors. Arch Otolaryngol Head Neck Surg 1991;117:189–193

Schuknecht HF, Allam AF, Murakami Y. Pathology of secondary malignant tumors of the temporal bone. Ann Otol Rhinol Laryngol 1968;77:5–22

Suryanarayanan R, Dezso A, Ramsden RT, Gillespie JE. Metastatic carcinoma mimicking a facial nerve schwannoma: the role of computerized tomography in diagnosis. J Laryngol Otol 2005;119:1010–1012

CHAPTER 33 Cochlear Malformations
Mohannad Ibrahim

Epidemiology

Congenital deafness accounts for 19% of hearing loss in the population. Bony anomalies associated with a congenital sensorineural hearing loss (SNHL) are fairly uncommon, representing approximately 16 to 20% of the cases of congenital SNHL. The remaining 80 to 84% of congenital SNHL is due to membranous malformation in which the bony architecture of the inner ear is normal. Anomalies of the otic capsule can involve a single structure or the entire capsule. Cochlear malformation can result from an arrest of embryogenesis, abnormal development, or genetic defects that may result in distinctive cochlear anomalies.

Clinical Features

A family history of hearing loss is present in only 12% of the population. Profound SNHL is the presenting symptom that is usually discovered in early childhood, although some patients might have mild, progressive hearing loss. Associated anomalies of the middle ear and cerebrospinal fluid leak/perilymph leak are frequently encountered in these patients (24%). There is an increased risk of recurrent meningitis in patients with congenital temporal anomalies.

Pathology

The inner ear consists of a membranous labyrinth surrounded by an osseous labyrinth or otic capsule. The maturation of the membranous and osseous labyrinth has three main phases: development (4th to 8th week), growth (8th to 16th week), and ossification (16th to 24th week). The development of the sensory epithelium within the membranous labyrinth occurs simultaneously with growth and ossification (8th to 24th week). The membranous labyrinth differentiates from ectodermal primordium, the otic placode, which arises along the lateral aspect of the neural tube. The auditory pit develops from the otic placode during the 4th week, which then invaginates to become the otocyst during the 5th week. The otocyst then divides into a cochlear and vestibular pouch, both of which will later form the various components of the mature membranous labyrinth. The otic capsule develops as a cartilaginous condensation of mesenchyme around the otic vesicle between the 4th and 8th weeks of gestation. Ossification of the otic capsule to form the osseous labyrinth begins at 15 weeks.

The modiolus (Latin for "hub of the wheel") is the central bony axis about which the spiral canal of the osseous cochlea winds 2½ to 2¾ turns. The interscalar septa are consistently visible on imaging as thin bony projections that connect the inner wall of the cochlea to the modiolus. The osseous spiral lamina of the cochlea is the thin bony shelf that projects from the modiolus and supports the organ of Corti, separating the scala tympani and scala vestibule of cochlea.

Many classifications of the inner ear dysplasia relied mainly on the concept of arrest at different stages of embryologic development. Jackler et al classified four types of cochlear anomalies: complete aplasia (3rd week arrest), cochlear aplasia (late 3rd week arrest), common cavity (4th week arrest), cochlear hypoplasia (6th week arrest), and incomplete partition of the cochlea. Sennaroglu et al added

118

many other cochlear anomalies to his classification scheme, which was also dependent on the concept of developmental arrest at different stages of embryogenesis. Papsin et al suggested multiple distinct anomalous paths of cochlear development that might arise during otic placode development. Absence of cochleovestibular development will result in Michel's anomaly. Subsequently, anomalous development of the otocyst might result in a common cavity, or a little more development can occur and a cystic cochleovestibular anomaly can result. A separate anomalous development of the otocyst can result in a cochlea in which there is complete development of the otocyst with distinct cochlear and vestibular elements; however, there is significantly diminished growth in one or both elements, resulting in cochlear hypoplasia. Often, a narrow internal auditory canal accompanies this anomaly. The Mondini anomaly represents a divergent path of anomalous development of the otocyst, in which the differentiated cochlear and vestibular elements are present but with incomplete partitioning within the cochlea and enlargement of the vestibular aqueduct.

Treatment

If the contralateral ear is normal, the patient will be able to hear, and no treatment is indicated. The absolute requirements for cochlear implantation are the presence of cochlea (either normal or malformed) and cochlear nerve. Cochlear implantation is expected to provide some clinical benefit regardless of the degree of dysplasia.

Imaging Findings

Cochlear aplasia, or Michel's anomaly, is the most severe form of cochlear dysplasia and is characterized by complete absence of the inner ear structures. The region of the otic capsule normally occupied by the cochlea and vestibule is replaced by dense bony labyrinthine lesions. The common cavity is characterized by confluence of the cochlea, vestibule, and semicircular canals in a saccular defect or cavity. This entity accounts for 26% of cochlear malformations. Cystic cochleovestibular anomaly accounts for less than 2% of all congenital labyrinthine lesions. It is characterized by an enlarged ductus reunion with a cystic featureless cochlea and an enlarged vestibule. Cochlear hypoplasia is a malformation of the inner ear characterized by a small deformed cochlea that has a single turn or less. This disorder accounts for approximately 15% of all cochlear anomalies. The Mondini malformation is the most common inner ear malformation, accounting for 55% of otic capsule dysplasia. There is an overuse of this term to describe many of the inner ear anomalies. However, based on the original description by Carol Mondini in 1791, it is characterized by a shortened cochlea with 1½ turns: a normal basal turn and a cystic apex in place of the distal 1½ turns, an enlarged vestibule with normal semicircular canals, and an enlarged vestibular aqueduct (**Fig. 33–1, Fig. 33–2, Fig. 33–3, Fig. 33–4,** and **Fig. 33–5**).

IMAGING PEARLS _____

- The presence of the cochlear promontory in postmeningitis labyrinthine ossificans helps to differentiate this entity from labyrinthine aplasia.
- An aberrant course of the facial nerve is identified in 16% of patients with cochleovestibular anomalies.

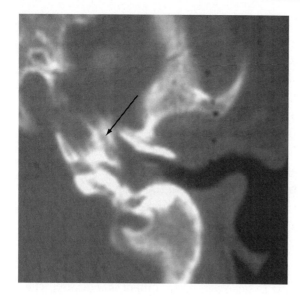

Figure 33–1 Michel's anomaly. Axial computed tomography (CT) of the temporal bone shows a bony absence of the inner ear (*arrow*), which is indicative of Michel's aplasia. This is thought to be due to a lack of formation of the otic vesicle. (Case courtesy of Doug Philips, M.D., University of Virginia.)

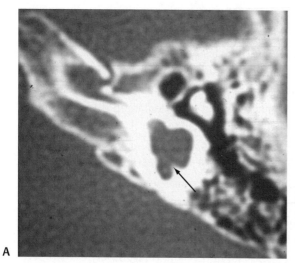

A

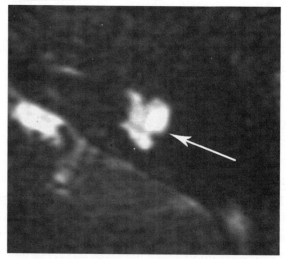

B

Figure 33–2 A common cavity. **(A)** Axial CT through the temporal bone shows a cystic cavity (*arrow*) in the inner ear, which is characteristic of a common cavity malformation. **(B)** Axial heavily T2-weighted magnetic resonance imaging performed in the same patient as in **A** shows fluid within the common cavity malformation (*arrow*). The internal auditory canal (IAC) is not formed, indicating absence of the cochlear nerve. This is a contraindication for cochlear implantation.

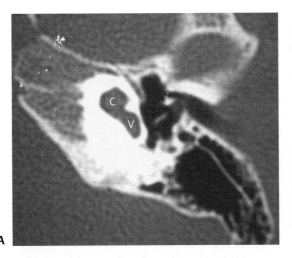

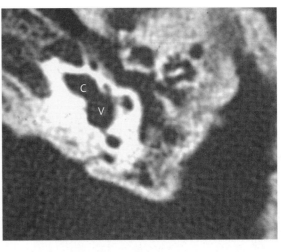

A   B

Figure 33–3 Severe cochlear hypoplasia. **(A,B)** Axial CT performed in two separate patients shows early separation of the cochlea (c) and vestibule (v). Although the vestigial structures still communicate, there is evidence of differentiation into two separate structures.

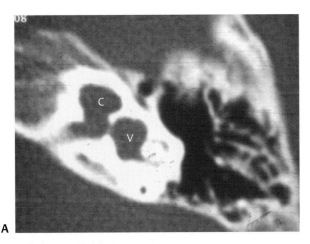

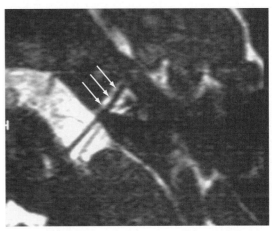

A   B

Figure 33–4 Moderate cochlear hypoplasia. **(A)** Axial CT shows complete separation of the cochlea (c) and vestibule (v). However, there is no internal differentiation of the cochlea with fusion of all turns. **(B)** Axial heavily T2-weighted imaging shows the cochlear nerve (*arrows*) to be present in the IAC. The caliber of the nerve is normal and the patient underwent a successful cochlear implantation.

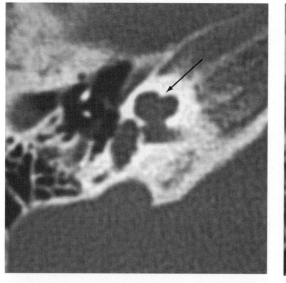

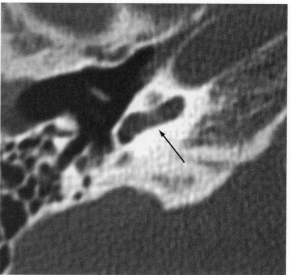

A

B

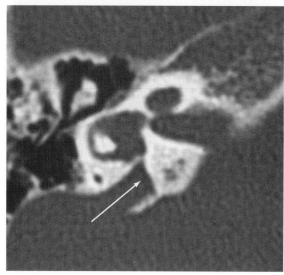

C

Figure 33–5 A Mondini malformation. **(A)** Axial CT shows fusion of the apical and middle turns (*arrow*) of the cochlea. **(B)** Axial CT shows that the basal turn (*arrow*) is intact. **(C)** Axial CT at the level of the petrous apex shows enlargement of the vestibular aqueduct (*arrow*). The enlarged vestibular aqueduct was described in association with the fusion of the apical and middle turns of the cochlea in the patient originally described by Mondini.

Suggested Readings

Jackler RK, Luxford WM, House WF. Congenital malformations of the inner ear: a classification based on embryogenesis. Laryngoscope 1987;97:2–14

Jackler RK, Hwang PH. Enlargement of the cochlear aqueduct: fact or fiction? Otolaryngol Head Neck Surg 1993;109:14–25

Nair SB, Abou-Elhamd KA, Hawthorne M. A retrospective analysis of high resolution computed tomography in the assessment of cochlear implant patients. Clin Otolaryngol 2000;25:55–61

Papsin BC. Cochlear implantation in children with anomalous cochleovestibular anatomy. Laryngoscope 2005;115(1 pt 2 suppl 106):1–26

Park AH, Kou B, Hotaling A, Azar-Kia B, Leonetti J, Papsin B. Clinical course of pediatric congenital inner ear malformations. Laryngoscope 2000;110:1715–1719

Semanogly L, Isil S. A new classification for cochleovestibular malformation. Laryngoscope 2002;112: 2230–2241

Mohannad Ibrahim

Epidemiology

Anomalies of the semicircular canals (SCCs) may coincide with the presence of a morphologically normal cochlea. These anomalies are often associated with other anomalies of the inner ear; thus they should be considered as part of diffuse inner ear malformations. SCC anomalies are often bilateral, with one side is more affected than the other. There is a high association between SCC aplasia and the CHARGE association (coloboma of the eye, congenital heart defects, choanal atresia, developmental and growth retardation, genital hypoplasia, and ear anomalies/or deafness). Isolated aplasia of the posterior semicircular duct has been described in patients with Wartenberg and Alagille syndrome.

Clinical Features

The most common presenting symptom is sensorineural hearing loss, even when the cochlea is normal on imaging. Conductive hearing loss is often present due to associated oval window atresia and ossicular chain malformation. Dizziness is present in only 19% of the patients. A few patients complain of Tullio phenomenon, which is dizziness upon hearing loud noises.

Pathology

The vestibule is the largest cavity of the bony labyrinth. The saccule and utricle reside within the vestibule, with the saccule located anteroinferiorly anchored to the spherical recess, and the utricle located posterosuperiorly anchored to the elliptical recess. The utriculosaccular duct connects the saccule and the utricle together. On the posterior wall of the utricle reside five openings for the three semicircular ducts (the superior and posterior canals have a common crus). Each of the SCCs is an arc of approximately two thirds of a full circle, oriented at right angles to each other. The superior SCC is in an oblique sagittal plane, approximately perpendicular to the long axis of the petrous bone. The vestibule is considered abnormally large when the ratio of the transverse diameter of the vestibule in the axial plane to the inner diameter of the lateral semicircular canal exceeds 1:2.

The development of the semicircular canals is completed between the 19th and 22nd week of gestation. Its development starts at the 4th week, along with the other inner ear structures, from the vestibular anlage. It begins as two fingerlike extensions from the utricular side of the otic vesicle. Between weeks 4 and 8, the membranous labyrinth has three subdivisions: the saccule with the cochlear duct (pars inferior), the utricle with its SCCs (pars superior), and the endolymphatic duct system. Embryologically, the pars superior, semicircular canals, and utricle are phylogenetically older than the pars inferior, cochlea, and saccule. As a result, developmental malformations are more common in the neolabyrinth (cochlea and saccule) than in the paleolabyrinth (SCCs and utricle). Complete maturation of the SCC occurs at about mid-gestation, with the superior SCC completed first and the lateral SCC completed last.

In general, the severity of any inner ear anomaly is believed to depend on the timing of the developmental insult. Because the lateral SCC is the last to form, it is probably more prone to developmental anomalies. Given the sequence of inner ear embryogenesis, an insult to the inner ear between weeks 8 and 20 may interrupt formation of the membranous SCCs while sparing the membranous cochlear duct. However, many cases of the agenesis of the SCC with a morphologically normal cochlea could not be easily explained based on embryogenic arrest, because the membranous vestibular labyrinth begins to develop earlier than the membranous cochlear duct.

A more selective, probably genetic, disorder of SCC development might explain this anomaly, particularly in syndromic cases. Specific genetic mutations linked to SCC anomalies have been found in mice. The detections of similar mutations in humans might help to guide genetic counseling in the future.

Treatment

Mild, sporadic SCC dysplasia may have minimal clinical impact and require no treatment in unilateral involvement. In syndromic SCC dysplasia the affected ear will never hear and the patient might benefit from cochlear implantation.

Imaging Findings

CT

Computed tomography (CT) is the modality of choice for evaluating patients with semicircular canal anomalies. The most common anomaly of the SCC is a dilated lateral SCC forming a single cavity with the vestibule. The posterior and superior SCC may be normal, dilated, or hypoplastic. The cochlea can be normal, or more commonly abnormal with incomplete apical and middle turn partition. Other cochlear anomalies include cochlear aplasia, cochlear hypoplasia, or a common cavity. There might be associated oval window atresia or anomalies of the middle ear ossicles, especially in syndromic cases. An anomalous course of the facial nerve canal is often encountered, with some of these patients having clinical symptoms of facial nerve dysfunction, especially in patients with the CHARGE association. A short and broad lateral SCC is encountered less often. Anomaly of the common crus of the superior and posterior SCC is commonly seen. It can be abnormally enlarged or even absent. Aplasia of the SCC is commonly seen in association with other syndromes, mainly the CHARGE association. The cochlea can be normal, or more commonly there are associated cochlear anomalies, cochlear hypoplasia, or Mondini dysplasia (**Fig. 34–1, Fig. 34–2, Fig. 34–3,** and **Fig. 34–4**).

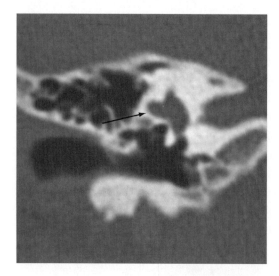

Figure 34–1 Coronal computed tomography (CT) shows dysplasia of the lateral semicircular canal (*arrow*). The canal is shorter and thicker than normal.

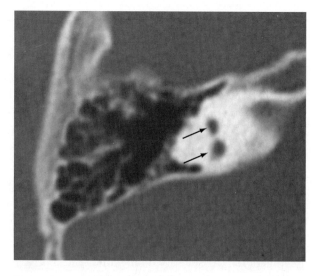

Figure 34–2 Axial CT obtained through the superior semicircular canal demonstrates dysplasia of the both anterior and posterior crux (*arrows*). The caliber of the canal is larger than normal and the distance between the anterior and posterior crux is decreased.

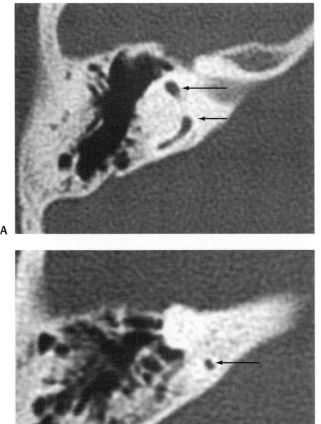

A

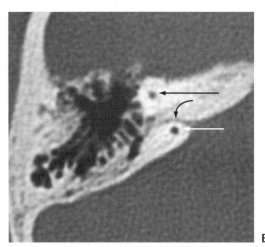

B

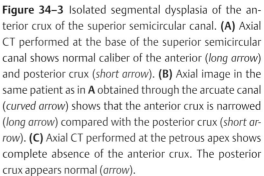

C

Figure 34–3 Isolated segmental dysplasia of the anterior crux of the superior semicircular canal. **(A)** Axial CT performed at the base of the superior semicircular canal shows normal caliber of the anterior (*long arrow*) and posterior crux (*short arrow*). **(B)** Axial image in the same patient as in **A** obtained through the arcuate canal (*curved arrow*) shows that the anterior crux is narrowed (*long arrow*) compared with the posterior crux (*short arrow*). **(C)** Axial CT performed at the petrous apex shows complete absence of the anterior crux. The posterior crux appears normal (*arrow*).

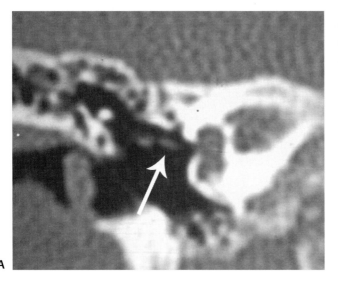

A

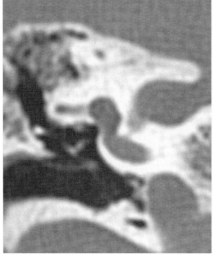

B

Figure 34–4 Complete semicircular canal aplasia. **(A)** Coronal CT obtained through the level of the oval window shows complete absence of the lateral and superior semicircular canals. The absence of the lateral semicircular canal has resulted in the tympanic segment of the facial nerve "floating" in the middle ear cavity (*arrow*). Compare this to the normal appearance **(B)**.

MRI

The semicircular canals can be visualized on magnetic resonance imaging (MRI), and semicircular canal dysplasias can be detected. Reformations are helpful in assessing these anomalies. MRI often requires more sedation than is required with multidetector CT, which has a shorter acquisition time. As a result, when given the choice between the two modalities, referring physicians often choose CT.

IMAGING PEARLS _____

- Both of the coronal and axial planes are required to confirm oval window atresia and anomalous facial nerve course.
- Anomalies of the SCC are commonly associated with cochlear anomalies and should be considered part of a diffuse inner ear malformation.

Suggested Readings

Davidson HC, Ric Harnsberger H, Lemmerling MM, et al. MR evaluation of vestibulocochlear anomalies associated with large endolymphatic duct and sac. AJNR Am J Neuroradiol 1999;20:1435–1441

Jackler RK, Luxford WM, House WF. Congenital malformations of the inner ear: a classification based on embryogenesis. Laryngoscope 1987;97:2–14

Satar B, Mukherji SK, Telian SA. Congenital aplasia of the semicircular canals. Otol Neurotol 2003;24:437–446

Yu KK, Mukherji S, Carrasco V, Pillsbury HC, Sores CG. Molecular genetic advances in semicircular canal abnormalities and sensorineural hearing loss: a report of 16 cases. Otolaryngol Head Neck Surg 2003;129:637–646

CHAPTER 35 Large Vestibular Aqueduct Syndrome

Mohannad Ibrahim

Epidemiology

Large vestibular aqueduct syndrome is one of the most common anomalies seen in patients with congenital sensorineural hearing loss (SNHL), and is the most commonly identified radiologic anomaly on cross-sectional imaging of the inner ear. Valvassori and Clemis first described this anomaly in 1978; they reported their conventional polytomographic findings in 50 patients and named this condition the large vestibular aqueduct syndrome (LVAS). It has been reported to be bilateral in 55 to 94% of cases. LVAS is typically associated with other malformations of the inner ear. The most common malformation is a modiolar deficiency, which lies along the spectrum of a Mondini malformation. In fact, in Mondini's original description of the malformation, the child was also noted to have an enlarged vestibular aqueduct. Hence there is some debate as to whether these entities should even be considered separate. Overall, it is common to consider LVAS a separate entity from a Mondini malformation. Isolated LVAS without involvement of the rest of the inner ear structures is uncommon, present in 0 to 14% of the patients.

Clinical Features

Patients might be asymptomatic, or present with a sensorineural hearing loss that may be mild to profound. The hearing loss can be fluctuant and progressive, often with sudden, stepwise onset or progression, sometimes secondary to trigger activities such as the Valsalva maneuver, minor head injury, common cold, scuba diving, and others.

Anatomy and Embryology

The endolymphatic duct and sac are the nonsensory components of the membranous labyrinth. The endolymphatic duct extends in the vestibular aqueduct from the utricle medially to the endolymphatic sac laterally, which is located in the epidural space of the posterior fossa. The distal end of the sac overlaps the adjacent sigmoid sinus in 40% of the population. Embryologically, there is a progressive nonlinear growth of the vestibular aqueduct throughout gestation. The growth of the vestibular aqueduct does not decline or reach a maximum size during fetal life, and it continues to grow postnatally until age 3 or 4 years. A nonspecific early insult might result in persistence of the fetal form of the endolymphatic duct and a short, wide vestibular aqueduct. However, recent investigations suggest that LVAS may be due to an acquired deformity as opposed to a congenital malformation. In adults, the average width of the vestibular aqueduct ranges from 0.4 to 1.0 mm.

Pathology

The mechanism by which LVAS causes a progressive SNHL is still unknown. Several possible mechanisms of cochlear damage have been proposed, including disruption of homeostasis secondary to reflux of hyperosmolar fluid from the endolymphatic sac into the inner ear, direct transmission of intracranial pressure to the inner ear via the large vestibular aqueduct injury caused by pressure effects, and susceptibility to minor trauma. Generally LVAS is nonfamilial; however, a genetic predisposition has been reported in a portion of the patients with LVAS, with most of the reported cases being sporadic. Recent reports suggested an autosomal recessive inheritance. LVAS may be associated with both nonsyndromic and syndromic forms of SNHL.

Treatment

Aside from behavior modification to limit trauma, no accepted treatment for this condition exists. Surgical occlusion and obliteration of the endolymphatic sac have been tried; however, the surgery has limited success.

Imaging Findings

CT

The defining morphologic feature of this condition is enlargement of the vestibular aqueduct measuring >1.5 mm in its mid-bony portion. As a general rule, LVAS is present when the bony vestibular aqueduct diameter is larger than the posterior semicircular canal or facial nerve canal diameter. Coexistent inner ear anomalies are common in LVAS, although the frequency with which these anomalies are reported to occur has been inconsistent among authors. It is generally seen in 84 to 100% of cases. Cochlear anomalies are the most common anomaly reported with LVAS and appear as a spectrum, ranging from subtle modiolar deficiency to gross dysplasia. Modiolar deficiency is the most frequent cochlear finding. Scalar asymmetry is commonly seen in conjunction with gross cochlear dysmorphism, both of which are also manifestations of cochlear dysplasia. Anomalies of the vestibule, particularly enlarge-

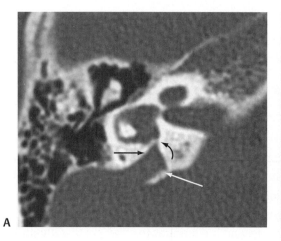

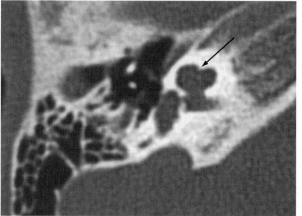

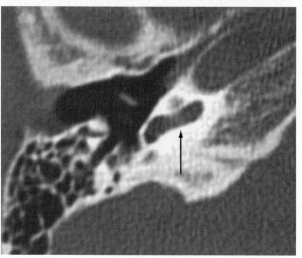

Figure 35–1 Large vestibular aqueduct syndrome. **(A)** Axial CT obtained through the petrous apex shows enlargement of the vestibular aqueduct (*straight arrows*). The distal portion of the vestibular aqueduct (*curved arrow*) is communicating with the common crus. **(B)** Axial CT performed through the oval window demonstrates absence of the modiolus with fusion of the apical and middle turns of the cochlea (*straight arrow*). **(C)** Axial CT obtained through the carotid canal shows a normal basal turn of the cochlea (*arrow*).

ment of the membranous vestibule, are quite common. Gross vestibular dysplasia and semicircular canal (SCC) abnormality are also part of the spectrum of associated vestibular anomalies (**Fig. 35–1**).

MRI

The magnetic resonance imaging (MRI) findings are best detected on heavily weighted T2 sequences and are similar to computed tomography (CT) with enlargement of the vestibular aqueduct and underlying endolymphatic sac. Modiolar deficiency can be detected on MRI. Overall, CT is performed more commonly than MRI since the scan time is shorter, which results in less sedation requirements. However, both modalities can be used to make the diagnosis.

IMAGING PEARLS

- Cochlear and vestibular anomalies are commonly associated with LVAS.
- The vestibular aqueduct diameter should not be larger than the adjacent posterior semicircular canal diameter.

Suggested Readings

Davidson HC, Harnsberger HR, Lemmerling MM, et al. MR evaluation of vestibulocochlear anomalies associated with large endolymphatic duct and sac. AJNR Am J Neuroradiol 1999;20:1435–1441

Lai CC, Shiao AS. Chronological changes of hearing in pediatric patients with large vestibular aqueduct syndrome. Laryngoscope 2004;114:832–838

Lo WWM, Daniels DL, Chakeres DW, et al. The endolymphatic duct and sac. AJNR Am J Neuroradiol 1997;18:881–887

Mafee MF, Charletta D, Kumar A, Belmont H. Large vestibular aqueduct and congenital SNHL. AJNR Am J Neuroradiol 1992;13:805–819

Pyle GM. Embryological development and large vestibular aqueduct syndrome. Laryngoscope 2000;110:1837–1842

Valvassori GE, Clemis JD. The large vestibular aqueduct syndrome. Laryngoscope 1978;88:723–728

CHAPTER 36 Internal Auditory Canal Stenosis/Atresia

Diana Gomez-Hassan

Epidemiology

An internal auditory canal (IAC) measuring less than 2 mm in vertical dimension by high-resolution temporal bone computed tomography (CT) is considered stenotic. Approximately 12% of patients with congenital sensorineural hearing loss have radiographic evidence of inner ear abnormalities including IAC stenosis. IAC stenosis without other abnormalities is extremely rare.

Clinical Features

Patients with IAC stenosis may present with congenital sensorineural hearing loss caused by aplasia of the vestibulocochlear nerve during development, but in very rare cases it can be asymptomatic.

Pathology

In addition to primary causes of IAC narrowing, osseous lesions such as an exostosis or an osteoma can cause secondary narrowing of the IAC. Also, underlying skeletal disease causing hypertrophy of the surrounding bone (Paget's disease or otosclerosis) can contribute to IAC stenosis. Hyperpneumatization of the petrous apex can also result in abnormal narrowed conditions.

Treatment

In most cases of congenital sensorineural hearing loss caused by IAC stenosis, hearing devices or cochlear implantation may not be helpful. In asymptomatic IAC stenosis, palliative IAC decompression of cochlear nerve can be considered if sudden onset of deafness occurs.

Imaging Findings

CT

An axial image obtained using 1- to 1.5-mm, thick-section, high-resolution CT is the best method to detect IAC stenosis. The normal range of the IAC diameter is 2 to 8 mm, with an average of 4 mm. The literature defines IAC stenosis when the diameter is less than 2 mm (**Fig. 36–1, Fig. 36–2,** and **Fig. 36–3**).

MRI

Magnetic resonance imaging often provides additional information regarding the presence and caliber of the seventh and eighth nerves but is less useful in defining the osseous anatomy of the canal wall.

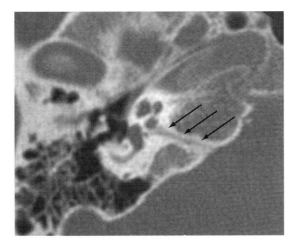

Figure 36–1 Axial computed tomography (CT) of the right ear demonstrates a stenotic internal auditory canal (*arrows*).

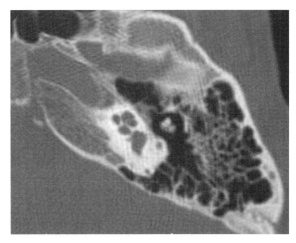

Figure 36–2 Axial CT obtained through the left temporal bone in the same patient illustrated in Figure 36–1 demonstrates atresia of the internal auditory canal.

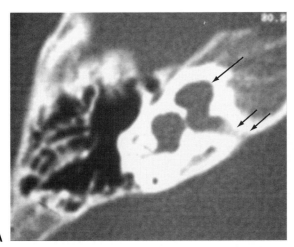

A

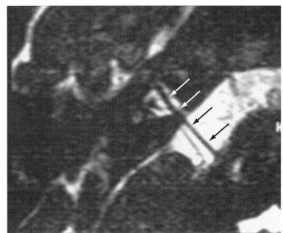

B

Figure 36–3 (A) Axial CT demonstrates cochlear hypoplasia (*large arrow*) associated with stenosis of the internal auditory canal (*small arrows*). **(B)** This was a candidate for a cochlear implant who underwent a CISS (0.7 mm) study to determine if the cochlear nerve was present. The study shows bony stenosis of the internal auditory canal. The cochlear nerve is present (*small arrows*). Based on visualization of the cochlear nerve, the patient underwent a successful cochlear implant.

IMAGING PEARLS

- Congenital IAC stenosis occurs when the diameter is less than 2 mm.
- High-resolution T2-weighted MRI may be helpful to evaluate the caliber of the cochlear nerve in patients with hearing loss who have a stenotic IAC.
- Decompression may only be helpful when acute onset of symptoms occurs.

Suggested Readings

Baek SK, Chae SW, Jung HH. Congenital internal auditory canal stenosis. J Laryngol Otol 2003;117:784–787

Cho YS, Na DG, Jung JY, Hong SH. Narrow internal auditory canal syndrome: parasagittal reconstructions. J Laryngol Otol 1997;123:1238–1239

Davis TC, Thedinger BA, Greene GM. Osteomas of the internal auditory canal: a report of two cases. Am J Otol 2000;21:852–856

Shelton C, Luxford WM, Tonokawa LL, Lo WWM. House contraindication to cochlear implants. Otolaryngol Head Neck Surg 1989;100:227–231

Valvassori GE, Pierce RH. The normal internal auditory canal. Am J Roentgenol 1964;92:1232–1241

CHAPTER 37 Oval Window Aplasia/Hypoplasia

Suresh K. Mukherji

Epidemiology

Congenital absence (atresia, aplasia) of the oval window is a known cause of congenital hearing loss. The prevalence of this disease has increased due to advances in computed tomography (CT) that permit routine imaging at or below 1.0-mm-thick sections. Oval window atresia is known to be associated with external auditory canal atresia. However, this potentially correctable cause of congenital hearing loss may still be missed. Patients typically present in the first decade of life with a mixed or conductive hearing loss associated with congenital hearing loss.

Embryology

The embryogenesis of oval window atresia is related to development of the second branchial arch structures and the nerve associated with second arch (facial nerve). The lenticular process of the incus, stapes suprastructure, and facial nerve are all derived from the second arch. The oval window arises from the otic capsule, but the oval window does not form unless the footplate of the stapes is fully developed. There are currently two theories that attempt to explain oval window atresia. One theory directly associates abnormal formation of the oval window to the development of the facial nerve. The tympanic and descending portions of the facial nerve become anteriorly and inferiorly displaced. This places the nerve between the stapes anlage and oval window and prevents induction of the oval window. The second theory is that the atresia is due to underdevelopment of the second branchial arch, which results in anterior shifting of second arch structures.

Treatment

The potential treatment of oval window aplasia is surgical. However, the surgical outcomes have been variable. In addition, the malposition of the facial nerve places this nerve at greater risk during surgery. Thus the detection of oval window aplasia in the presence of external auditory canal atresia may prevent some patients from undergoing surgical repair at some institutions.

Imaging Findings

CT

The imaging finding of oval window atresia is the presence of a bony plate in the expected region of the oval window. Partial absence has also been reported. The associated findings include inferomedial malposition of the facial nerve, malformed incus, and dysplastic or absent stapes (**Figs. 37–1** and **Fig. 37–2**).

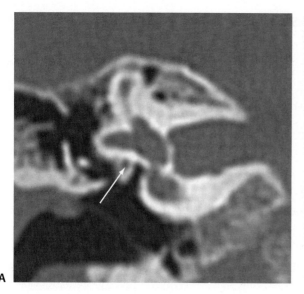
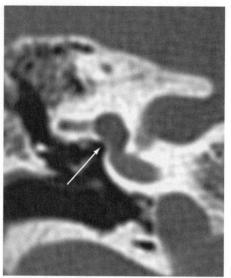

A   B

Figure 37–1 Oval window aplasia. Coronal computed tom-ography (CT) is performed through the midportion of the vestibule of the right window. **(A)** A patient with isolated oval window aplasia. Note the bony covering over the ex-pected location of the oval window (*arrow*). This lack of bony resorption is characteristic of aplasia of the oval window. Compare this with the normal appearance of the oval win-dow (*arrow*) **(B)**.

MRI

There is no defined need for magnetic resonance imaging (MRI) to evaluate oval window atresia. The small size of the structure and susceptibility artifacts of air in the middle cavity and the bone surround-ing the inner make detailed evaluation of the oval window difficult.

IMAGING PEARLS _____

- Oval window aplasia can be diagnosed only if the persistent bony plate is seen in two planes.
- Oval window hypoplasia may be isolated or may occur in association with other inner ear anoma-lies.
- Submillimeter thick sections are required for ensuring the most accurate diagnosis.
- Multiplanar reconstructions may be helpful to make the diagnosis.

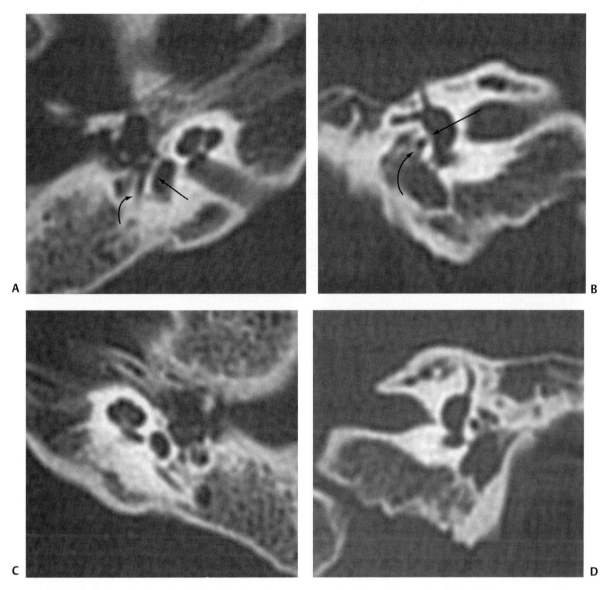

Figure 37–2 Bilateral oval window aplasia with anomalous course of the facial nerve and hypoplastic middle ear cavity. **(A)** Axial and **(B)** coronal CT performed through the right temporal bone demonstrates a bony plate covering the oval window (*straight arrow*), which is indicative of aplasia of the oval window. The course of the facial nerve (*curved arrow*) is well below and is located at the level of the midportion of the expected location of the oval window. The middle ear cavity is underdeveloped (M). **(C,D)** Similar findings are seen on the opposite side as well.

Suggested Readings

Booth TN, Vezina LG, Karcher G, Dubovsky EC. Imaging and clinical evaluation of isolated atresia of the oval window. AJNR Am J Neuroradiol 2000;21:171–174

Zeifer B, Sabini P, Sonne J. Congenital absence of the oval window: radiologic diagnosis and associated anomalies. AJNR Am J Neuroradiol 2000;21:322–327

CHAPTER 38 Cholesterol Granuloma of the Petrous Apex
Gaurang V. Shah

Epidemiology

Cholesterol granuloma of the petrous apex was accepted as a distinct entity only in the mid-1980s. The most accepted pathogenesis is the obstruction-vacuum hypothesis. Mucosal engorgement occludes the narrow petrous apex outflow tracts. Absorption of trapped gas leads to a vacuum with development of negative pressure, which results in the breakdown of a few blood vessels, with pooling of blood. Anaerobic breakdown of blood products results in production of cholesterol crystals, which incites a foreign-body reaction leading to sterile inflammatory conditions, which erode the bone and lead to further hemorrhage and cholesterol formation.

An alternate exposed bone-marrow hypothesis stipulates that budding mucosa invades and replaces bone marrow of the petrous apex in young adulthood. Hemorrhage from exposed marrow leads to mucosal swelling and obstruction of draining pathways, leading to anaerobic breakdown of pooled blood into cholesterol. According to this theory, obstruction of outflow is secondary to hemorrhage from marrow and not the primary trigger for the hemorrhage. Recurrent hemorrhages lead to further enlargement and expansion of the cyst containing cholesterol crystals, forming an expansile mass at the petrous apex.

For the lesions at the petrous apex, the terms *cholesterol cyst* and *cholesterol granuloma* are interchangeable; although for middle ear and mastoid region, a granuloma is preceded by inflammation or infection, whereas a cyst is not.

Clinical Features

Cholesterol granulomas can be classified as nonaggressive or aggressive based on clinical symptoms and radiologic features. Nonaggressive types are asymptomatic and often incidentally diagnosed. The aggressive types are more common. There are three dominant clinical patterns based on involvement of adjacent structures.

In the first type, sensorineural hearing loss and tinnitus are the most common presenting symptoms. Vertigo and dizziness are other common presenting conditions. It seems that dysfunction of cranial nerve VIII is the most typical presenting disability, and involvement of the internal auditory canal radiologically is a common finding. The second type is related to a cholesterol granuloma located in the superior part of the petrous apex, in which temporal headache and facial pain are the principal presenting symptoms. This type is attributed to compression of the dura of the middle and posterior fossa. In the third type, there is involvement of the trigeminal and abducens nerves, indicating compression of the Meckel cave region. Recurrent otitis media is less common but sometimes a unique clinical feature, attributed to compression of the eustachian tube by the cyst.

Pathology

A cholesterol granuloma contains hemorrhagic debris as brownish fluid containing cholesterol crystals. Red blood cells, hemosiderin, blood vessels, chronic inflammatory cells, and multinucleate giant cells are also visualized. The granuloma is outlined by thick fibrous connective tissue.

Treatment

The surgical route for accessing the lesion depends on the degree of loss of presurgical hearing acuity, the size of the mass, and the relationship between the lesion and petrous temporal anatomy including the jugular bulb. Drainage and stent placement by a transtemporal approach is the most traditional treatment. The transsphenoidal and posterior fossa approaches are also utilized in some settings. However, an extended middle cranial fossa approach with extradural removal of the mass and obliteration of lesion cavity decreases the rate of recurrence.

Presurgical evaluation by both a computed tomography (CT) scan and magnetic resonance imaging (MRI) are considered essential for presurgical planning. Patients with asymptomatic cholesterol cyst should have lifelong follow-up for progression because enlargement might occur even after years of stability.

Imaging Findings

CT

Computed tomography is very well suited to evaluate the boundary of the lesion, which is predominantly intraosseous. A cholesterol granuloma has a characteristic appearance of an expansile petrous apex mass with thinned out margins. The matrix of lesion is hypodense on soft tissue windows but the evaluation is more useful on bone windows. Uniformly thinned out or erosive margins are highly characteristic.

The most important contribution of CT scan is depiction of an anatomic relationship with temporal bone structures such as the jugular bulb, internal acoustic canal, otic capsule, and air cell tracts. The thickness of the wall between a cholesterol cyst and infralabyrinthine or infracochlear air cells greatly aids in planning the surgical route; a thick wall makes the infracochlear approach much harder.

Other important features to evaluate on CT include involvement of the cochlea, sphenoid bone, facial nerve, carotid canal, and cavernous sinus, and any prior postoperative changes (**Fig. 38–1**).

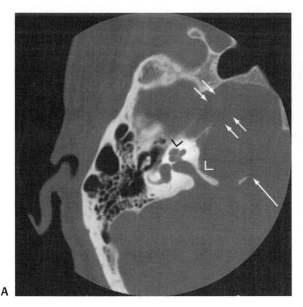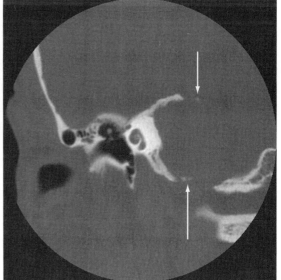

A   B

Figure 38–1 Computed tomography (CT) findings of a cholesterol cyst. **(A)** Axial image shows an expansile, lytic mass at the right petrous apex (*large arrow*). There is uniform remodeling of the bone with erosion of bony septa. Erosion of the carotid canal is also seen (*small arrows*). There is mild remodeling of internal auditory canal, but the cochlea is spared (*arrowhead*). **(B)** Coronal CT shows an expansile focal mass at the level of cochlea with erosion of remodeled bony wall of the lesion (*arrows*). The middle ear cavity is completely normal.

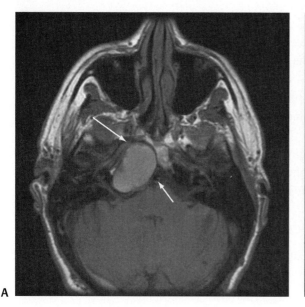

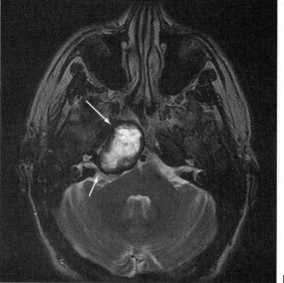

A

B

Figure 38–2 Magnetic resonance imaging (MRI) findings of cholesterol cyst. **(A)** Axial T1-weighted MRI shows the lesion as homogeneously hyperintense (*large arrow*). The mass expands in to the right side of prepontine cistern and basisphenoid at the expected location of cranial nerve VI and abuts the basilar artery (*small arrow*). **(B)** T2-weighted axial MRI shows a predominantly hyperintense mass (*large arrow*). The peripheral areas of low T2 signal likely represent hemosiderin-laden macrophages. There is mild deformity of the ventral surface of the pons due to the mass. There is remodeling of the anterior wall of the internal acoustic canal with underlying mass effect of the VII/VIII nerve complex (*small arrow*).

MRI

In conjunction with CT, MRI is virtually diagnostic for cholesterol granuloma. A short T1 signal due to cholesterol formation and a long T2 signal due to the presence of fluid are characteristic for cholesterol granuloma, which appears bright on almost all MRI sequences. Sometimes a peripheral ring of low signal is seen on T2-weighted images. This is due to the presence of hemosiderin-laden macrophages in the fibrous wall, which is quite thick. Due to the ability of MRI to image soft tissue structures like the fibrous wall, the margins of cholesterol granuloma appear much thicker on MRI than on CT scan, which shows only a thinned out bony margin. Due to its inherently superior soft tissue resolution, MRI is also better in evaluating intracranial soft tissue structures like the vestibulocochlear nerve, facial nerve, trigeminal nerve, cochlea, Meckel cave, dural venous sinuses, and dural reflections (**Fig. 38–2**).

The characteristic MRI appearance also helps to differentiate cholesterol granuloma from congenital cholesteatoma, petrous apex arachnoid cyst, neuroma, and chondrosarcoma. Less frequent lesions such as a thrombosed giant aneurysm or rare hydrated mucocele may prove to be diagnostically challenging.

On MRI following surgical drain, there is a characteristic loss of bright T1 signal with persistent high T2 signal. This is due to loss of cholesterol crystals.

IMAGING PEARLS _____

- An expansile petrous apex mass with a thinned out bony wall with or without bone erosion is the characteristic appearance of a cholesterol granuloma on CT.
- An expansile petrous apex mass that appears hyperintense on both T1- and T2-weighted images is characteristic appearance for cholesterol granuloma on MRI. It is also most helpful in assessing intracranial extension and postsurgical follow-up.
- Both MRI and CT are also essential for planning the surgical approach to the lesion. Lifelong follow-up is recommended, even for indolent nonaggressive cholesterol granuloma.

- Other etiologies to be considered in the differential diagnosis of expansile petrous apex masses on CT include arachnoid cyst, epidermoid cyst, intraosseous neuroma, and giant aneurysm. Thrombosed aneurysm and hydrated mucocele may be a potential diagnostic dilemma on MRI.

Suggested Readings

Brackmann DE, Toh EH. Surgical management of petrous apex cholesterol granulomas. Otol Neurotol 2002;23:529–533

Chang P, Fagan PA, Atlas MD, Roche J. Imaging destructive lesions of the petrous apex. Laryngoscope 1998;108:599–604

Curtin HD, Som PM. The petrous apex. Otolaryngol Clin North Am 1995;28:473–496

Graham MD, Kemink JL, Latack JT. The giant cholesterol cyst of the petrous apex: a distinct clinical entity. Laryngoscope 1985;95:1401–1406

Greenberg JJ, Oot RF, Wismer GL, et al. Cholesterol granuloma of the petrous apex, MR and CT evaluation. AJNR Am J Neuroradiol 1988;9:1205–1214

Jackler RK, Cho M. A new theory to explain the genesis of petrous apex cholesterol granuloma. Otol Neurotol 2003;24:96–106

Mosnier I, Cyna-Gorse F, Grayeli AB. Management of cholesterol granulomas of the petrous apex based on clinical and radiologic evaluation. Otol Neurotol 2002;23:522–528

Thorne MC, Gebarski SS, Telian SA. Rapid expansion in a previously indolent cholesterol cyst: a need for lifelong follow-up. Otol Neurotol 2006;27:124–126

CHAPTER 39 Acute Labyrinthitis
Vaishali Phalke

Epidemiology

Acute labyrinthitis is an inflammatory process of the membranous labyrinth. The inflammatory response may be secondary to infections—bacterial, viral, or leutic—or may be secondary to trauma or autoimmune processes. There can be different routes for infection to reach the cochlea. It may be a complication of bacterial meningitis (meningogenic), in which infection can spread into the inner ear from the cochlear aqueduct. Infection can spread into the labyrinth also through a hematogenous route (hematogenic) via the cochlear vasculature. The most common cause is due to viral infections, though measles, mumps, tuberculosis, syphilis, and other bacterial infections can also spread via the hematogenous route. Posttraumatic labyrinthitis occurs either due to prior iatrogenic injury, from middle ear surgery, or due to prior injury. Labyrinthitis may be a complication of acute otomastoiditis (tympanogenic) with infection spreading from the middle ear cavity via the oval or round windows or through direct invasion of the bony labyrinth through a fistula in the lateral semicircular canal.

Clinical Features

Sudden sensorineural hearing loss and vertigo are common. Vertigo may be severe enough to cause nausea and vomiting. There are no associated auditory or central nervous system symptoms. This helps to differentiate labyrinthitis from cerebellar infarction, vestibular schwannoma, and Meniere disease, which can also present with sensorineural hearing loss. The disease may manifest as a single attack, or a patient may have multiple attacks. The acute phase may last for days to weeks, with generally complete recovery occurring around 6 months. There may be associated otitis media. Milder attacks of shorter duration of vertigo may occur in patients with multiple attacks.

Pathology

The most common bacterial pathogens are *Haemophilus influenza, Neisseria meningitidis, Streptococcus pneumoniae, Escherichia coli, Proteus, Listeria monocytogenes,* and *Mycobacterium tuberculosis.* Viral labyrinthitis is the most common cause of delayed hydrops syndrome. The pathology can be divided into three stages. During the acute stage, bacteria and leukocytes appear first in the perilymphatic spaces along with a serofibrinous exudate. In the later fibrous stage, there is formation of granulation tissue that is composed of hypertrophic fibroblasts and increasing angiogenesis. The ossification stage is demonstrated by newly formed disorganized woven bone.

Treatment

Acute labyrinthitis due to bacterial meningitis is usually treated with antibiotics. Steroids may be administered to help reduce meningeal inflammation. When labyrinthitis is secondary to viral infections, treatment is symptomatic in the form of vestibular suppressants, antiemetics, and good hydration.

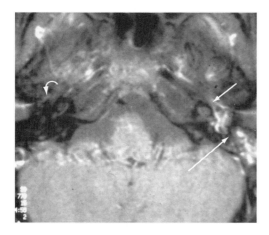

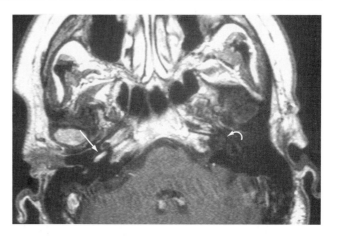

Figure 39–1 Fat-suppressed contrast-enhanced T1-weighted magnetic resonance imaging (MRI) shows an abnormally enhancing cochlea (*small arrows*) secondary to acute otitis media (*large arrow*). These findings are typical for acute labyrinthitis (cochleitis). Note the normal appearance of the uninvolved cochlea on the contralateral side (*curved arrow*).

Figure 39–2 Contrast-enhanced T1-weighted imaging performed in a patient with acute labyrinthitis shows marked enhancement of the basal turn of the right cochlea (*straight arrow*). Note the normal appearance of the cochlea on the uninvolved left side (*curved arrow*).

Imaging Findings

CT

There are no specific imaging findings in acute labyrinthitis. Tympanogenic causes may result in opacification of the middle ear cavity. Computed tomography (CT) may be used to exclude associated findings such as semicircular canal fistulas or tegmen defects, which result in direct communication of the labyrinth with the middle ear or cerebrospinal fluid (CSF), respectively.

MRI

There is diffuse enhancement of the cochlea and vestibule. Tympanogenic acute labyrinthitis may be associated with fluid in the middle ear cavity. Meningogenic causes may be associated with abnormal enhancement of the meninges (**Fig. 39–1** and **Fig. 39–2**).

IMAGING PEARLS _____

- Magnetic resonance imaging (MRI) is the modality of choice.
- Precontrast T1 images are important to exclude hemorrhage or the presence of proteinaceous material within the labyrinth.
- Other causes of sensorineural hearing loss such as vestibular schwannoma and cerebellar infarction can be excluded by MRI.

Suggested Readings

Gulya A. Infections of the labyrinth. In: Bailey B, ed. Head and Neck Surgery–Otolaryngology, 2nd ed. Philadelphia: Lippencott-Raven, 1998:2137–2151

Mark AS, Fitzgerald D. Segmental enhancement of the cochlea on contrast-enhanced MR: correlation with the frequency of hearing loss and possible sign of perilymphatic fistula and autoimmune labyrinthitis. AJNR Am J Neuroradiol 1993;14:991–996

Nemzek WR, Swartz JD. Temporal bone: inflammatory disease. In: Som PM, Curtin HD, eds. Head and Neck Imaging, 4th ed. St. Louis: Mosby, 2003:1173–1229

Paparella MM, Suguira S. The pathology of suppurative labyrinthitis. Ann Otol Rhinol Laryngol 1967;76:554–586

CHAPTER 40 Labyrinthitis Ossifications

Ashok Srinivasan

Epidemiology

Also termed "ossifying labyrinthitis" and "labyrinthine ossification," labyrinthitis ossificans (LO) refers to the chronic pathologic ossification of the labyrinth and cochlea from an infectious, inflammatory, traumatic, or surgical insult. Although the most common cause of LO is suppurative bacterial labyrinthitis, other causes include viral labyrinthitis, autoimmune inner ear disease, advanced otosclerosis, labyrinthine artery occlusion, leukemia, and temporal bone tumors. Since bacterial labyrinthitis primarily involves children, LO is observed mainly in the pediatric population.

Clinical Features

Due to involvement of the labyrinth, bilateral sensorineural hearing loss is the most common clinical presentation of LO. Patients with LO may also suffer from vertigo of variable severity, sometimes requiring labyrinthectomy. There is gradual deterioration of hearing after the inciting event, which can be infectious meningitis, trauma, or surgery.

Pathology

Suppurative infection of the membranous labyrinth causes a cascade of inflammatory reactions that result in initial fibrosis followed by ossification. Bone formation can be seen as early as 2 months following the inciting event. On gross pathologic examination, there is new bone formation noted in the membranous labyrinth. Microscopic examination reveals fibroblast proliferation in the initial stages followed by prominent osteoblastic activity. Scala tympani of the basal turn of the cochlea is the most frequently involved area of ossification in LO resulting from any cause.

Treatment

Cochlear implantation is used for treating the sensorineural loss due to LO. It is important to recognize bilateral cochlear LO because bilaterality is a detriment to cochlear implantation.

Imaging Findings

CT

Nonenhanced high-resolution computed tomography (CT) of the temporal bone reveals a spectrum of findings in LO varying from hazy areas of increased density resulting from fibrosis within the fluid spaces of the membranous labyrinth to focal or complete obliteration of the fluid spaces by new bone formation. This can result in a complete "white-out" appearance of the membranous labyrinth. The modiolus can appear prominent. Contrast-enhanced CT has no role in the diagnosis or characterization of LO (**Fig. 40–1, Fig. 40–2, Fig. 40–3,** and **Fig. 40–4A**).

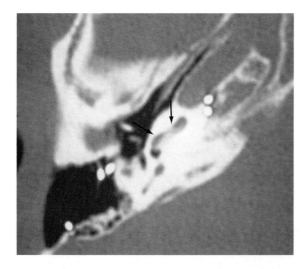

Figure 40–1 Axial computed tomography (CT) of the temporal bone shows early labyrinthitis ossificans (LO) involving the basal turn of the cochlea. Note the increased attenuation involving the basal turn of the cochlea (*arrows*), indicating early ossification.

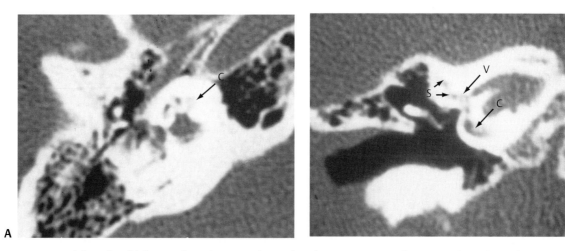

Figure 40–2 **(A)** Axial and **(B)** coronal CT of a more advanced LO demonstrating ossification involving the cochlea (C), vestibule (v), and semicircular canals (S).

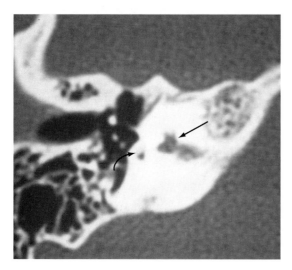

Figure 40–3 Axial CT of the temporal bone obtained in a patient with advanced LO. The cochlea is nonvisualized ("white-out"). Only a remnant of the cochlear canal (*straight arrow*) indicates the expected location of the cochlea. There is also advanced ossification of the vestibule (*curved arrow*).

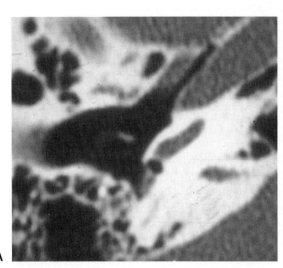

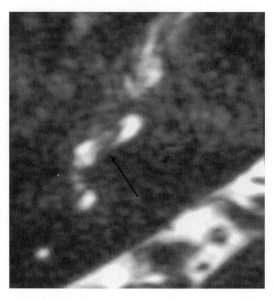

A

B

Figure 40–4 Greater sensitivity for detecting disease with magnetic resonance imaging (MRI) than with CT. **(A)** Axial CT performed through the temporal bone shows a normal-appearing basal turn of the cochlea. **(B)** Axial heavily weighted T2 image shows a focal lesion (*arrow*) located in the basal turn of the cochlea that was not seen on the CT. This information is important for otologists prior to cochlear implantation, as it indicates that they may need to remove these areas of fibro-osseous obliteration to successfully insert the electrode

MRI

On T2-weighted magnetic resonance imaging (MRI), fibrosis is visualized as intermediate or low signal areas within the high signal fluid spaces of the membranous labyrinth. There may also be apparent enlargement of the modiolous. With progression of LO, there is progressive encroachment and replacement of high signal fluid spaces by low signal new bone. On postgadolinium T1-weighted images, there is usually segmental or holo-labyrinthine enhancement in the infectious stage of the disease due to active labyrinthitis. This abnormal enhancement may variably persist into the ossifying stages of LO (**Fig. 40–4B**).

IMAGING PEARLS _____

- The basal turn of the cochlea is the most frequently involved area in LO.
- It is important to recognize cochlear versus noncochlear LO because cochlear involvement makes treatment more complex.
- Advanced bilateral cochlear LO may contraindicate cochlear implantation.
- Differential diagnosis includes labyrinthine schwannoma (in the early stages of LO where there is labyrinthine enhancement) and cochlear otosclerosis (does not encroach on membranous labyrinth even in the healing phase).

Suggested Readings

Becker TS, Eisenberg LS, Luxford WM, House WF. Labyrinthine ossification secondary to childhood bacterial meningitis: implications for cochlear implant surgery. AJNR Am J Neuroradiol 1984;5:739–741

Casselman JW, Kuhweide R, Ampe W, Meeus L, Steyaert L. Pathology of the membranous labyrinth: comparison of T1- and T2-weighted and gadolinium-enhanced spin-echo and 3DFT-CISS imaging. AJNR Am J Neuroradiol 1993;14:59–69

Casselman JW, Majoor MH, Albers FW. MR of the inner ear in patients with Cogan syndrome. AJNR Am J Neuroradiol 1994;15:131–138

deSouza C, Paparella MM, Schachern P, Yoon TH. Pathology of labyrinthine ossification. J Laryngol Otol 1991;105:621–624

Green JD Jr, Marion MS, Hinojosa R. Labyrinthitis ossificans: histopathologic consideration for cochlear implantation. Otolaryngol Head Neck Surg 1991;104:320–326

Hoffman RA, Brookler KH, Bergeron RT. Radiologic diagnosis of labyrinthitis ossificans. Ann Otol Rhinol Laryngol 1979;88:253–257

Jackler RK, Dillon WP, Schindler RA. Computed tomography in suppurative ear disease: a correlation of surgical and radiographic findings. Laryngoscope 1984;94:746–752

Suga F, Lindsay JR. Labyrinthitis ossificans. Ann Otol Rhinol Laryngol 1977;86:17–29

Swartz JD, Mandell DM, Faerber EN, et al. Labyrinthine ossification: etiologies and CT findings. Radiology 1985;157:395–398

Weissman JL, Kamerer DB. Labyrinthitis ossificans. Am J Otolaryngol 1993;14:363–365

CHAPTER 41 Petrous Apicitis
Diana Gomez-Hassan

Epidemiology

Petrous apicitis is a rare infection of the petrous apex of the temporal bone that occurs as a result of the spread of middle ear or mastoid infection. In the past, this disease was more widespread but became much more uncommon with the introduction of antibiotics. The diagnosis may be considered in patients with a chronic suppurative ear infection that is associated with deep ipsilateral pain.

Clinical Features

The entity of petrous apicitis has become synonymous with Gradenigo syndrome. This results from advanced suppurative otitis media that spreads to the petrous apex and involves adjacent intracranial structures. The clinical findings consist of middle ear infection with otorrhea, retro-orbital pain, and a sixth nerve palsy resulting in diplopia. The sixth nerve palsy is due to involvement of the sixth nerve as it extends through the Dorello canal, which is formed in part by the petroclinoid ligament. The retro-orbital pain may be due to compression or irritation of the gasserian ganglion of the trigeminal nerve (trigeminal ganglionitis). Advanced disease may involve cranial nerves II, III, VII, IX, and X.

Patients may complain of vague or indistinct symptoms that delay diagnosis. Headaches, atypical facial pain, mixed hearing loss, vertigo, eustachian tube dysfunction, and middle ear effusion are common complaints. Facial nerve dysfunction is less common, except in advanced lesions. Hearing loss and vestibular complaints may be caused by eighth nerve involvement in the internal auditory canal or by direct extension of the process into the bony labyrinth.

Pathology

Petrous apicitis is believed to occur when organisms, typically pseudomonads, become trapped within the complex air cells of the petrous apex. The spread to the petrous apex is thought to arise from direct extension of advanced suppurative otitis media. This typically is thought to occur in pneumatized air cells; however, this is controversial. Potential complications include meningitis, cerebritis, intracranial abscess (epidural or intracerebral), and venous sinus thrombosis.

Treatment

Once the diagnosis of petrous apicitis is made, intravenous antibiotics are considered first. In severe, potentially life-threatening cases, aggressive therapy such as surgical drainage is needed.

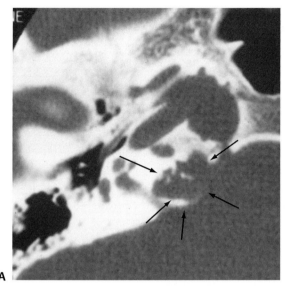
A

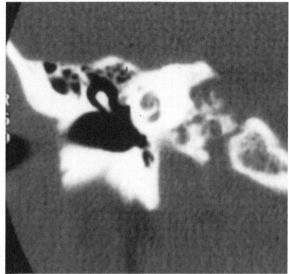
B

Figure 41–1 Petrous apicitis. **(A)** Axial and **(B)** coronal computed tomography (CT) of the right temporal bone shows the characteristic scalloped bone erosion (*arrows*) seen in petrous apicitis. This may be due to an osteitis or osteomyelitis of the bone.

Imaging Findings

CT

Thin-section high-resolution bone algorithm computed tomography (CT) scanning is most useful in the delineation of bone destruction in the apex. Temporal bone features diagnostic of petrous apicitis on CT scan include opacification of the mastoid air cell system, specifically within the pneumatized petrous apex, enhancement of the cavernous sinus, and bony erosion within the petrous apex. With contrast, cavernous sinus enhancement also may occur (**Fig. 41–1**).

MRI

Magnetic resonance imaging (MRI) can be complementary to CT in characterizing the lesion within the petrous apex. In acute apicitis, high-resolution MRI with gadolinium demonstrates a low-intensity signal on T1-weighted images, shows a hyperintense signal on T2-weighted images, and has ring enhancement with gadolinium. MRI can help to distinguish this entity from others that occur in the petrous apex, including congenital or primary cholesteatoma, cholesterol granuloma, primary mucocele, schwannoma, meningioma, chondroma, chondrosarcoma, or metastatic neoplasms. Discernment of pathologic processes in this area and evaluation of their extent is critical in diagnosis and preoperative planning (**Fig. 41–2, Fig. 41–3,** and **Fig. 41–4**).

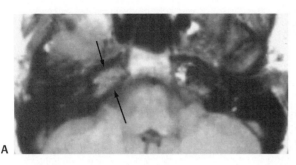

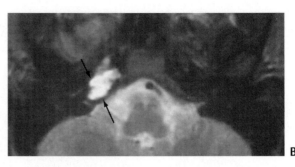

Figure 41–2 Mucosal thickening of the petrous apex. **(A)** Axial T1-weighted (T1W) and **(B)** T2-weighted (T2W) magnetic resonance imaging (MRI) of the temporal bone shows intermediate T1W signal and high T2W signal (*arrows*). These findings are indicative of mucosal thickening and do not necessarily indicate the presence of petrous apicitis. The diagnosis of petrous apicitis can be determined only based on the patient's presenting symptoms

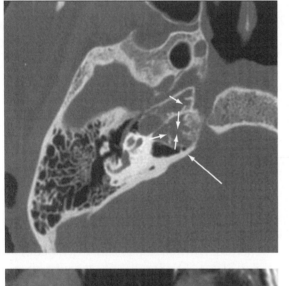

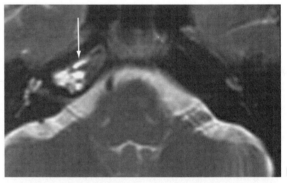

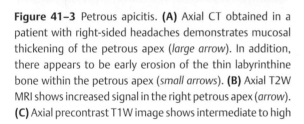

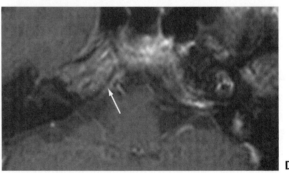

Figure 41–3 Petrous apicitis. **(A)** Axial CT obtained in a patient with right-sided headaches demonstrates mucosal thickening of the petrous apex (*large arrow*). In addition, there appears to be early erosion of the thin labyrinthine bone within the petrous apex (*small arrows*). **(B)** Axial T2W MRI shows increased signal in the right petrous apex (*arrow*). **(C)** Axial precontrast T1W image shows intermediate to high signal in the petrous apex indicating proteinaceous material (*arrow*). **(D)** Axial postcontrast T1W images shows enhancement of the abnormality in the petrous apex (*arrow*). The patient was started on antibiotic therapy and dramatically improved and was given a presumptive diagnosis of petrous apicitis.

(Courtesy of Christine Glastonbury, MD.)

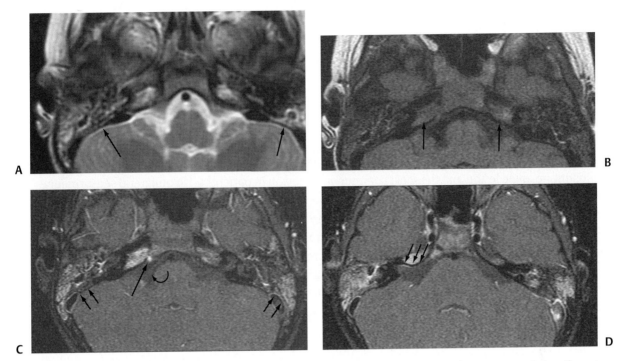

Figure 41–4 A 7-year-old girl with a history of bilateral otomastoiditis and right sixth nerve palsy. **(A)** Axial T2W image shows mucosal thickening involving the mastoid air cells bilaterally (*arrows*). **(B)** Noncontrast T1W images show symmetric intermediate signal involving the petrous apices (*arrows*). **(C)** Contrast-enhanced T1W with fat-suppression shows asymmetric enhancement of the right petrous apex (*large straight arrow*) with a small focal area of enhancement in the region where the sixth nerve enters below the petroclinoid ligament (Dorello canal) (*curved arrow*). There is also symmetric enhancement of the mastoid air cells (*small arrows*). **(D)** Axial contrast-enhanced T1W image with fat-suppression also show linear dural enhancement along the anterior portion of the right internal auditory canal (*arrows*).

(Courtesy of Nancy Fischbein, MD.)

IMAGING PEARLS

- MRI shows low T1 signal, high T2 signal, and rim enhancement with the petrous apex.
- CT imaging demonstrates osseous erosion of the petrous apex and opacification of the pneumatized portion of the petrous pyramid but also opacification in the mastoid air cells and middle ear cavity.

Suggested Readings

Chole RA, Donald PJ. Petrous apicitis. Clinical considerations. Ann Otol Rhinol Laryngol 1983;92(6 pt 1):544–551

Curtin HD, Som PM. The petrous apex. Otolaryngol Clin North Am 1995;28:473–496

Nemzek WR, Swartz JD. Temporal bone: inflammatory disease. In: Som PM, Curtin HD, eds. Head and Neck Imaging, 4th ed. St. Louis: Mosby 2003:1173–1229

CHAPTER 42 Vestibular Schwannoma
Vaishali Phalke

Epidemiology

Acoustic neuroma of the eighth cranial nerve (vestibular schwannoma) is, by far, the most common cerebellopontine angle lesion and the most common mass lesion in patients with unilateral sensorineural hearing loss. It arises from the Schwann cells that wrap the vestibulocochlear nerve. It may arise in the internal auditory canal, porus acusticus, or in the internal auditory canal–cerebellopontine angle (IAC–CPA) cistern. It accounts for 8 to 10% of all intracranial tumors and 60 to 90% of all IAC-CPA tumors. Peak age of presentation is 40 to 60 years, though it may be seen in children with neurofibromatosis-2 (NF2). The tumor is slightly more common in females, though intracanalicular tumor may be more common in males. In NF2 patients, acoustic schwannomas are bilateral in 96%.

Clinical Features

Vestibular schwannoma usually presents with unilateral sensorineural hearing loss. Other common presentations include tinnitus, disequilibrium, and decreased speed discrimination. If these tumors are large, then trigeminal or facial neuropathy or even involvement of lower cranial nerves, cerebellar signs, and rarely even hydrocephalus and subarachnoid hemorrhage may occur. The duration of hearing loss before diagnosis is about 3 to 4 years; large tumors with brainstem compression often present with a shorter duration of symptoms and in younger patients.

Pathology

These tumors are slow-growing benign lesions arising from the vestibular portion of the eighth nerve at the oligodendrocyte–Schwann cell junction. Most tumors grow at the rate of 0.02 to 0.2 cm per year. A small percentage of tumors may grow faster, up to 1 cm or more per year.

They are encapsulated and arise eccentrically from the nerve originating in the nerve sheath. Histologically, these lesions are composed of differentiated neoplastic Schwann cells in a collagenous matrix. There are two main histologic spindle cell types: Antoni A tissue, which has a tendency to form palisades; and Antoni B cells, which are less cellular and more loosely arranged and may contain clusters of lipid-laden cells. There is no necrosis, but intramural cysts and rarely hemorrhage within Antoni B tissue may be present. There is strong diffuse expression of S-100 protein.

Treatment

Microsurgery with total resection of small tumors yields good functional preservation of the facial nerve. Hearing preservation is best when the tumor is less than 2 cm and does not invade the internal auditory canal fundus or cochlear aperture. Though there is considerable variation in the approach used, translabyrinthine resection of a large tumor is performed if no hearing preservation is possible. If tumor is intracanalicular, then a middle cranial fossa approach is used, and a suboccipital retrosigmoid approach is used when a cerebellopontine angle component is present. In the case of large acoustic neuromas, subtotal removal and subsequent radiosurgery is one option for maintaining cranial nerve function and long-term tumor growth control.

Imaging Findings

The overall appearance of a majority of acoustic schwannomas is that of an ice cream cone or mushroom, with a spherical IAC-CPA component centered at the acoustic porus and funnel-shaped extension into the IAC. The acute angle formed between the tumor and bone helps to differentiate schwannoma from the second most IAC-CPA tumor—meningioma. A small percentage of tumors may be entirely intracanalicular where they fill the IAC and have a convex medial margin.

CT

Bony changes are seen in larger acoustic schwannomas where tumors arising from the intracanalicular portion cause focal erosion of and flaring of the porus acusticus. There is a difference of 2 mm or more in canal height when compared with the normal side, a shortening of the posterior wall of the canal of more than 3 mm, and downward displacement of the crista falciformis. The tumor is generally isodense to the cerebellum, though it may be slightly hyperdense, hypodense, or of mixed density. Calcification is rare, and generally on contrast administration enhancement is homogeneous and dense.

MRI

Magnetic resonance imaging (MRI) is the study of choice for detecting vestibular schwannomas. Tumors are generally hypo- to isointense relative to the pons; and on postgadolinium T1-weighted images the sensitivity to detect an acoustic schwannoma is nearly 100%, with tumors enhancing strongly. Intramural cysts and hemorrhage may be present in larger tumors, with smaller tumors being generally homogeneous. On T2-weighted imaging, tumors are mildly hyperintense relative to the pons and iso- to hypointense to cerebrospinal fluid (CSF). Thus high-resolution T2-weighted imaging may be used as a screening tool where smaller tumors appear as an ovoid filling defect in the high signal CSF of IAC. On this high-resolution study it may be even possible to identify the nerve of origin of the smaller tumors. Involvement of the cochlear aperture or IAC fundus should be noted on imaging because it has

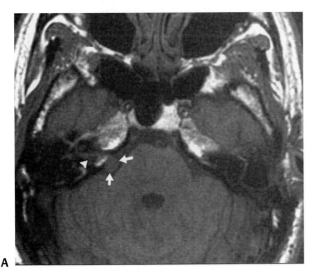
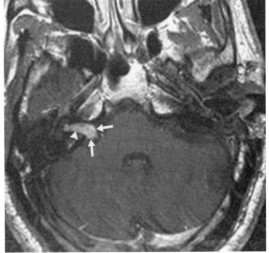

Figure 42–1 Magnetic resonance imaging (MRI) of vestibular schwannoma. **(A)** Axial precontrast T1-weighted image through the region of internal auditory canal shows a isointense mass in the region of right cerebellopontine angle (*white arrows*), with a funnel-shaped extension into the in- ternal auditory canal (*white arrowhead*). **(B)** Axial postgadolinium T1-weighted image at the same level as in **A** shows homogeneous enhancement of the mass in the right internal auditory canal–cerebellopontine angle (IAC-CPA).

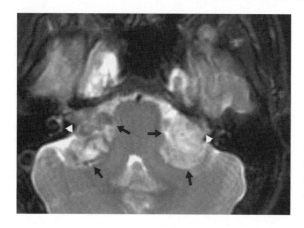

Figure 42–2 Bilateral acoustic schwannomas in neurofibromatosis-2 (NF2). Axial T2-weighted image through region of internal auditory canal shows large bilateral masses slightly hyperintense to the pons (*black arrows*) with funnel shaped extensions into the internal auditory canals (*white arrowheads*). When there are bilateral acoustic schwannomas, think of NF2.

a negative impact on hearing preservation surgery. Larger tumors may have mixed signal intensity due to the presence of cysts and hemorrhage. They may cause mass effect on the brainstem, where there may be edema and compression and displacement of the fourth ventricle. Giant tumors may also cause hydrocephalus, though it is extremely rare for them to herniate into the middle cranial fossa, unlike a meningioma (**Fig. 42–1** and **Fig. 42–2**).

IMAGING PEARLS

- High-resolution T2-weighted MRI can be used as a screening tool in a case of unilateral sensorineural hearing loss.
- When there are bilateral acoustic schwannomas, think of NF2.
- Differential diagnosis includes meningioma, epidermoid cyst, arachnoid cyst, facial nerve schwannoma, metastasis, and lymphoma,

Suggested Readings

Allen RW, Harnsberger HR, Shelton C. Low-cost high-resolution fast spin-echo MR of acoustic schwannoma: an alternative to enhanced conventional spin-echo MR? AJNR Am J Neuroradiol 1996;17:1205–1210

Curati WL, Graif M, Kingsley DP, et al. Acoustic neuromas: Gd-DTPA enhancement in MR imaging. Radiology 1986;158:447–451

Gruskin P, Carberry J. Pathology of Acoustic Tumors, Vol I: Diagnosis. Baltimore: University Park Press, 1979

Iwai Y. Surgery combined with radiosurgery of large acoustic neuromas. Surg Neurol 2003;59:283–289

Jackler RK, Pitts LH. Selection of surgical approach to acoustic neuroma. Otolaryngol Clin North Am 1992;25:361–387

Kasantikul V, Netsky MG, Glasscock ME III. Intracanalicular neurilemmomas: clinicopathologic study. Ann Otol Rhinol Laryngol 1980;89:29–32

Kim DG, Paek SH, Chi JG, et al. Mixed tumor of schwannoma and meningioma components in a patient with NF-2. Acta Neurochir (Wien) 1997;139:1061–1064

Lanser MJ, Sussman SA, Frazer K. Epidemiology, pathogenesis and genetics of acoustic neuromas. Otolaryngol Clin North Am 1992;25:499–520

Martuza RL, Eldridge R. Neurofibromatosis 2 (bilateral acoustic neurofibromatosis). N Engl J Med 1988;318:684–688

Matthies C, Samii M. Management of 1000 vestibular schwannomas (acoustic neuromas): clinical presentation. Neurosurgery 1997;40:1–10

Maya MM, Lo WWM, Kouvanlikaya I. Temporal bone tumors and cerebellopontine angle lesions. In: Som PM, Curtin HD, eds. Head and Neck Imaging, 4th ed. St. Louis: Mosby, 2003:1276–1286

Somers T, Casselman J, de Ceulaer G. Prognostic value of magnetic resonance imaging findings in hearing preservation surgery for vestibular schwannoma. Otol Neurotol 2001;22:87–94

Valvassori GE. The abnormal internal auditory canal: The diagnosis of acoustic neuroma. Radiology 1969;92:449–459

CHAPTER 43 Meningioma
Vaishali Phalke

Epidemiology

Meningioma is a benign neoplasm arising from the arachnoid cap cells in the internal auditory canal–cerebellopontine angle (IAC-CPA) cistern. These lesions account for approximately 15 to 18% of all primary intracranial tumors; 10% occur in the posterior fossa, 10% are multiple, and meningiomas along with schwannomas commonly occur in patients with neurofibromatosis-2 (NF2). Meningiomas are the second most common CPA-IAC tumor encountered after vestibular schwannoma and second most common primary intracranial tumor. Meningiomas are more common in females.

Clinical Features

These lesions are often incidentally detected, as patients are usually asymptomatic. If present, the symptoms are caused by compression of adjacent neural structures. Thus the patients may present with hearing loss, tinnitus, headache, or signs and symptoms related to trigeminal nerve. These lesions are common in the middle-aged and the elderly, with peak age of incidence being 60 years. When associated with NF2, they may be seen in children.

Pathology

Meningiomas arise from the arachnoid cap cells and not from the dura. These tumors are sharply circumscribed and unencapsulated. Approximately 60% of sporadic meningiomas are caused by inactivation of the NF2 tumor suppressor gene on chromosome 22. No causative genetic abnormality is known for the remaining 40%. Angiogenic factors such as fibroblast growth factor-2 (FGF-2), vascular endothelial growth factor (VEGF), and integrins are expressed in meningiomas. Meningiomas have also been found to have receptors to many hormones such as progesterone and prolactin and may express growth hormone.

The 2000 World Health Organization (WHO) classification grades meningiomas as benign (grade I), atypical (grade II), and anaplastic (grade III). There is a wide range of histologic subtypes with little bearing on prognostic outcome. These include those that have lobules of meningothelial cells; fibrous type with parallel, interlacing fascicles of spindle shaped cells; transitional with mixed type, which are characterized by onion bulb whorls and lobules; psammomatous type, which contains numerous small calcifications; and angiomatous comprising abundant vascular channels. There are miscellaneous forms that include microcystic, secretory, lymphoplasmocyte-rich meningioma, chondroid, clear cell, atypical, papillary, anaplastic, and rhabdoid meningiomas.

Treatment

Surgical resection is the treatment of choice. Radiotherapy may be used as adjuvant or as primary treatment if the lesions invade adjacent eloquent neurovascular structures.

Imaging Findings

CT

On non–contrast-enhanced computed tomography (CT), 69% of meningiomas are hyperdense, with calcifications seen in 25%. Although 10% of tumors may have inhomogeneous postcontrast enhancement, the majority (90%) of tumors shows strong uniform enhancement. Although the tumor may extend into the internal auditory canal, the canal is not expanded, but the bone may show hyperostotic or permeative changes.

MRI

The majority of meningiomas arising in the posterior fossa have a broad-based margin that abuts the adjacent dural surface. They grow eccentric to the porus acusticus and are hemispherical and may herniate into the middle cranial fossa. They tend to form an obtuse angle at the bone/tumor interface. These features sometimes aid in differentiating them from more common acoustic neuromas. Rare cases of meningiomas arising primarily within the internal auditory canal have been reported. It is difficult to differentiate them on imaging from vestibular schwannomas.

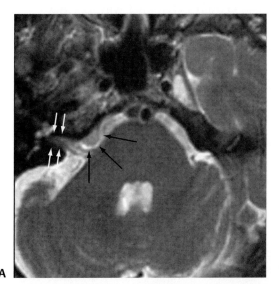

A

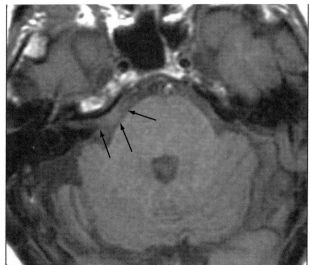

B

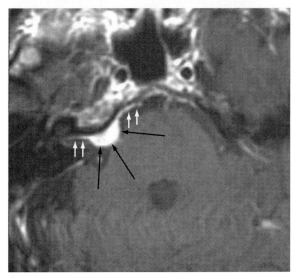

C

Figure 43–1 Magnetic resonance imaging (MRI) findings of meningioma. **(A)** Axial T2-weighted image shows a dural-based mass (*long arrows*) in the cerebellopontine angle cistern located eccentric to the porus acusticus (*short arrow*) that is slightly hyperintense to the pons. **(B)** Axial T1-weighted image shows isointense signal within the mass (*arrows*). **(C)** Axial contrast-enhanced T1-weighted image shows the mass (*long arrows*), which strongly enhances with an adjacent dural tail (*short arrows*).

Although 75% of meningiomas are isointense to gray matter on all sequences, 25% of masses may have internal necrosis, hemorrhage, and cyst formation. Most of the tumors show strong postgadolinium enhancement, but the enhancement may be heterogeneous in large tumors. Dural thickening, also referred to as a dural tail, may be seen in up to 60%. However, a dural tail is not specific for meningiomas, and when dural thickening extends into the internal auditory canal it can make differentiation from vestibular schwannoma extremely difficult. Peritumoral brain edema correlates with pial blood supply and angiogenic factors. High-grade meningiomas, such as anaplastic meningiomas, may invade the adjacent brain. Magnetic resonance imaging (MRI) spectroscopy is sometimes useful in the diagnosis of proliferative or malignant potential of meningiomas based on the cholesterol/creatinine ratio (**Fig. 43–1**).

Angiography

Generally the dural vessels supply the center and pial vessels supply the periphery. Prolonged vascular stain into venous phase with atrioventricular (AV) shunting is seen. The enlarged dural vessels may have a sunburst appearance. Preoperative embolization may be performed.

IMAGING PEARLS

- The presence of a dural tail can help differentiate a meningioma from a vestibular schwannoma.
- Differential diagnosis includes neurosarcoidosis, Lyme disease, tuberculosis; and idiopathic hypertrophic cranial pachymeningitis which may cause diffuse dural thickening and should be differentiated from en plaque or sessile meningiomas.

Suggested Readings

Aoki S, Sasaki Y, Machida T. Contrast-enhanced MR images in patients with meningioma: importance of enhancement of the dura adjacent to the tumor. AJNR Am J Neuroradiol 1990;11:935–938

Bello L, Zhang J, Nikas DC, et al. Alpha(v)beta3 and alpha(v)beta5 integrin expression in meningiomas. Neurosurgery 2000;47:1185–1195

Bohrer PS, Chole RA. Unusual lesions of the internal auditory canal. Am J Otol 1996;17:143–149

Brackmann DE, Bartels LJ. Rare tumors of the cerebellopontine angle. Otolaryngol Head Neck Surg 1980;88:555–559

Buetow MP, Buetow PC, Smirniotopoulos JG. Typical, atypical, and misleading features in meningioma. Radiographics 1991;11:1087–1106

Ciccarelli E, Razzore P, Gaia D. Hyperprolactinaemia and prolactine binding in benign intracranial tumours. J Neurosurg Sci 2001;45:70–74

Dowd CF, Halbach VV, Higashida RT. Meningiomas: the role of preoperative angiography and embolization. Neurosurg Focus 2003;15:E10

Ildan F, Tuna M, Gocer AP. Correlation of the relationships of brain-tumor interfaces, magnetic resonance imaging, and angiographic findings to predict cleavage of meningiomas. J Neurosurg 1999;91:384–390

Iwai Y, Yamanaka K, Yasui T. Gamma knife surgery for skull base meningiomas. The effectiveness of low dose treatment. Surg Neurol 1999;52:40–44

Lo W, Solti-Bohman L. Computed Tomography of the Petrous Bone and Posterior Fossa. New York: Marcel Dekker, 1987

Louis DN, Scheithauer BW, Budka H, et al. Meningiomas. In: Kleihues P, Cavenee WK, eds. Pathology and Genetics of Tumours of the Nervous System. Lyon, France: IARC Press, 2000:176–184

Pistolesi S, Fontanini G, Camacci T. Meningioma-associated brain oedema: the role of angiogenic factors and pial blood supply. J Neurooncol 2002;60:159–164

Rubenstein L. Tumors of the Central Nervous System, vol 6. Washington, DC: Armed forces Institute of Pathology, 1972

Schorner W, Schubeus P, Henkes H. Meningeal sign: a characteristic finding of meningiomas on contrast-enhanced MR images. Neuroradiology 1990;32:90–93

Shino A, Nakasu S, Matsuda M. Noninvasive evaluation of the malignant potential of intracranial meningiomas performed using proton magnetic resonance spectroscopy. J Neurosurg 1999;91:928–934

Valavanis A, Schubiger O, Hayek J. CT of meningiomas on the posterior surface of the petrous bone. Neuroradiology 1981;22:111–121

van Tilborg AA, Al Allak B, Velthuizen SC. Chromosomal instability in meningiomas. J Neuropathol Exp Neurol 2005;64:312–322

CHAPTER 44 Congenital Cholesteatoma of the Petrous Apex

Gaurang V. Shah

Epidemiology

The petrous apex has the shape of a three-sided pyramid. The base of this pyramid is formed from anterior to posterior by the carotid canal, the cochlea, the vestibule, and the semicircular canals. The internal auditory meatus divides this region into an anterior subdivision and a posterior subdivision, also known as the meato-labyrinthine area located between the meatus and the semicircular canals. However, only those cholesteatomas that involve the anterior subdivision are considered as true petrous apex cholesteatomas.

Congenital cholesteatoma of the petrous apex, also known as primary petrosal cholesteatoma, is believed to arise from persistent embryonic cell rests of epidermal tissue within the petrous bone. This is believed to happen during cephalic flexure of the embryonic head, when the mesenchyme that eventually forms the petrous temporal bone traps the epithelial cells from epithelial invagination, called a Seessel pocket between the third and fifth week of fetal life. This can lead to accumulation of epithelial cells and keratin.

Clinical Features

Congenital cholesteatomas of the petrous apex may occur without otorrhea and in an otherwise normal temporal bone. Headache is the commonest symptom. The apical cholesteatoma can extend toward the horizontal portion of the internal carotid artery, the trigeminal nerve, or the dura of the middle or posterior cranial fossa. The commonest presenting symptom is unilateral hearing loss, followed by palsies of cranial nerve VII. They can also present with vertigo or, rarely, with trigeminal symptoms.

Pathology

Congenital cholesteatoma is a solid lesion, lined with stratified squamous epithelium and filled with debris of pearly white whirls of keratin and cholesterol crystals that originate from progressive desquamation of the epithelium.

Treatment

Surgical excision is the treatment of choice. The translabyrinthine-transcochlear (transotic) approach, infralabyrinthine approach, and infracochlear approach represent the most direct surgical approaches. As opposed to surgical treatments for cholesterol granulomas and arachnoid cysts, these are aggressive approaches that require sacrifice of any residual hearing with or without transposition of the facial nerve.

The middle cranial fossa approach, which may allow for hearing preservation, may be performed in patients with good hearing and normal facial nerve function, but requires a craniotomy, affords poor access, and may involve traction on important neurologic structures with potential for injury.

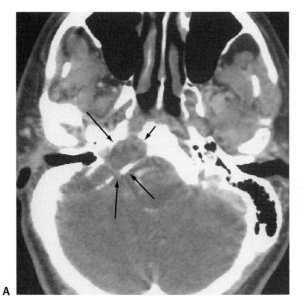
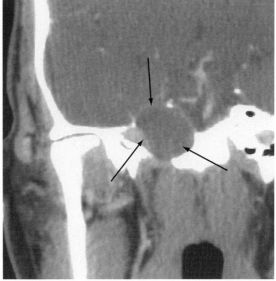

A

B

Figure 44–1 Computed tomography (CT) findings of congenital cholesteatoma of petrous apex. **(A)** Axial image shows an expansile, lytic mass in the right petrous apex with smooth margins and no contrast enhancement (*long arrows*). The lesion extends into the right petroclival fissure (*short arrow*). **(B)** Coronal CT shows an expansile focal mass at the level of the cochlea with thinning and demineralization of remodeled bony wall of lesion (*arrows*). (Courtesy of Amirsys.)

Imaging Findings

CT

Computed tomography (CT) delineates the expansile mass of congenital cholesteatoma and defines the extent of bone destruction. The margins are more often smooth than irregular; however, the latter is also reported. The mass is similar to cerebrospinal fluid (CSF) in density and does not exhibit any postcontrast enhancement. It is a unilateral process; however, bilateral cases have been reported. The anterior chamber of petrous apex is the site of origin, but the mass can expand toward the horizontal portion of the internal carotid artery laterally, the trigeminal nerve or the dura of the middle cranial fossa anteromedially, or the dura of posterior cranial fossa medially.

Other important features to evaluate on CT include involvement of the facial nerve or otic capsule and any prior postoperative changes.

Based on CT findings alone, a congenital cholesteatoma can be differentiated from solid tumors such as facial nerve neuroma, meningioma, glomus tumor, bone or cartilage tumor, chordoma, lymphoma, and epithelial tumor. However, cholesterol granuloma, arachnoid cyst, and mucocele may have similar CT findings (**Fig. 44–1**).

MRI

On magnetic resonance imaging (MRI), the expansile petrous apex mass may have low T1 signal, isointense to CSF, or somewhat intermediate signal, less intense than brain but more intense than CSF. The T2 signal is as intense as CSF. No enhancement is appreciated on postgadolinium studies. Bright signal on diffusion-weighted imaging is also reported and is considered an additional valuable tool for accurate diagnosis.

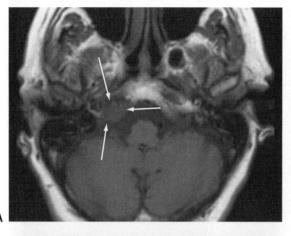

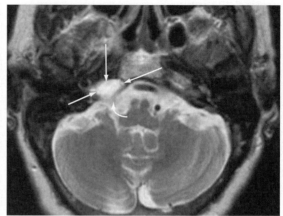

A

B

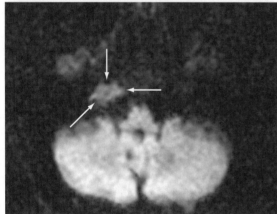

C

Figure 44–2 Magnetic resonance imaging (MRI) findings of congenital cholesteatoma of petrous apex. **(A)** Axial T1-weighted MRI shows an intermediate signal mass at the right petrous apex replacing normal high T1 signal of the bone marrow (*arrows*). The signal intensity of the lesion is higher than cerebrospinal fluid (CSF) but lower than brain parenchyma. **(B)** T2-weighted axial MRI shows a hyperintense expansile mass with signal intensity comparable to or higher than CSF (*arrows*). The inner margin of the mass encroaches on the inferior right cerebellopontine angle cistern (*curved arrow*). **(C)** Diffusion-weighted axial EPI image shows high signal mass in right petrous apex (*arrows*).

Due to its ability to visualize soft tissue structures, MRI is helpful in assessing the tumor margins, possible intracranial extension, and the relationship of the expansile mass with adjacent neural structures such as cranial nerve V and VII.

Magnetic resonance imaging is able to differentiate a low T1 signal congenital cholesteatoma from a high T1 signal cholesterol granuloma. An arachnoid cyst would have T1 and T2 signals similar to CSF. A rare petrous apex mucocele can have signal intensities similar to congenital cholesteatoma, but is considered to have a higher degree of variability in signal intensities on T1- and T2-weighted images (**Fig. 44–2**).

IMAGING PEARLS _____

- An expansile nonenhancing petrous apex mass, isodense to CSF with smooth margins, is characteristic CT appearance.
- MRI is most helpful in differentiating congenital cholesteatoma from cholesterol granuloma and arachnoid cyst, which can have similar features on CT. Bright signal on diffusion-weighted imaging is considered an important additional tool for accurate diagnosis.
- MRI is also useful for assessing the margins of the mass, possible intracranial extension, and the relationship with neural structures.
- Other etiologies to be considered in the differential diagnosis of expansile nonenhancing hypodense petrous apex masses on CT include cholesterol granuloma, arachnoid cyst, mucocele, and meningoencephalocele. Other less likely possibilities include chordoma, lymphoma, glomus tumor, meningioma, and facial nerve neuroma.

Suggested Readings

Chang P, Fagan PA, Atlas MD, Roche J. Imaging destructive lesions of the petrous apex. Laryngoscope 1998;108:599–604

Mafee MF, Kumar A, Heffner DK. Epidermoid cyst (cholesteatoma) and cholesterol granuloma of the temporal bone and epidermoid cysts affecting the brain. Neuroimaging Clin North Am 1994;4:561–578

Omran A, De Denato G, Piccirillo E, Leone O, Sanna M. Petrous bone cholesteatoma: management and outcomes. Laryngoscope 2006;116:619–626

Profant M, Steno J. Petrous apex cholesteatoma. Acta Otolaryngol 2000;120:164–167

Robert Y, Carcasset S, Rocourt N, Hennequin C, Dubrulle F, Lemaitre L. Congenital cholesteatoma of the temporal bone: MR findings and comparison with CT. AJNR Am J Neuroradiol 1995;16:755–761

Sheahan P, Walsh RM. Supralabyrinthine approach to petrosal cholesteatoma. J Laryngol Otol 2003;117:558–560

Yoshida T, Ito K, Adachi N, Yamasoba T, Kondo K, Kaga K. Cholesteatoma of the petrous bone: the crucial role of diffusion-weighted MRI. Eur Arch Otorhinolaryngol 2005;262:440–441

CHAPTER 45 Epidermoid
Vaishali Phalke

Epidemiology

Epidermoid or congenital cholesteatoma is a congenital benign slow-growing lesion. It occurs commonly in the posterior fossa, with the majority of epidermoid cysts occurring in the cerebellopontine angle–internal auditory canal (CPA-IAC) and in the fourth ventricle. Epidermoid is the third most common CPA-IAC lesion, with acoustic schwannomas and meningiomas being most common. It represents 0.2 to 1.8% of all intracranial tumors. Epidermoid cysts usually present between 20 and 70 years of age, with peak presentation being at 40 years.

Clinical Features

Epidermoids are slow-growing lesions that may remain clinically silent for many years. The principal presenting symptom is dizziness. Patients may also present with other symptoms such as headache, trigeminal (tic douloureux) and facial (hemifacial spasm) neuralgia, tinnitus, or sensorineural hearing loss depending on the location and growth pattern. Malignant degeneration of an epidermoid cyst is an extremely rare occurrence.

Pathology

This is a developmental lesion arising from the inclusion of ectodermal epithelial elements at the time of neural tube closure during the 3rd to 5th week of embryonic life, resulting in migration abnormalities of epiblastic cells. On gross pathology the lesion is pearly white with lobulated cauliflower-shaped surface features. On microscopy the cyst wall consists of stratified squamous epithelium. It grows in successive layers by desquamation from the cyst wall. The cyst contents are made up of solid crystalline cholesterol and keratinaceous debris without the presence of hair follicles, sebaceous glands, and fat, which helps to differentiate it from a dermoid.

Treatment

Complete surgical removal is the treatment of choice. However, total excision may be difficult if the lesion abuts or surrounds adjacent nerves and vessels.

Imaging Findings

CT

These lesions typically are low attenuation. The margins may be well demarcated or have irregular or scalloped margins. A homogeneously low-attenuation epidermoid with well-defined margins may be difficult to differentiate from an arachnoid cyst. The presence of high attenuation with the cyst can suggest the correct diagnosis. Dense epidermoids have been described.

MRI

Signal characteristics are similar to cerebrospinal fluid (CSF) on T1- and T2-weighted images. A dirty CSF signal has been described on T1-weighted images with moderately high signal also present on T2-weighted images. On fluid-attenuated inversion recovery (FLAIR) sequences, there is incomplete or absent attenuation and there is restricted diffusion on diffusion weighted imaging (DWI). No enhancement is seen on postgadolinium images. The presence of new enhancement should raise the suspicion of a squamous cell carcinoma arising from the epidermoid. Epidermoids may have irregular, infiltrative margins that may surround adjacent nerves and vessels. The cyst may insinuate into cisternal spaces and is located anterolateral or posterolateral to the brainstem (**Fig. 45–1** and **Fig. 45–2**).

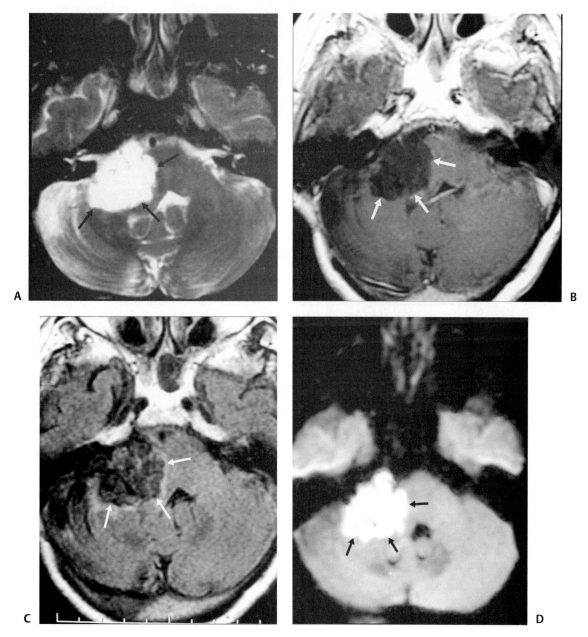

Figure 45–1 Magnetic resonance imaging (MRI) findings of an epidermoid. **(A)** Axial T2-weighted image shows a hyperintense mass (*arrows*) in the right cerebellopontine angle cistern with scalloped margins and mass effect on the surrounding structures. **(B)** On contrast-enhanced T1-weighted imaging, the mass (*arrows*) is predominantly isointense to cerebrospinal fluid (CSF) with no appreciable enhance-ment. **(C)** The fluid-attenuated inversion recovery (FLAIR) image shows incomplete fluid attenuation within the mass (*arrows*). **(D)** Restricted diffusion is present within the mass (*arrows*) on the diffusion-weighted images. Both FLAIR and diffusion images help to differentiate an epidermoid from an arachnoid cyst.

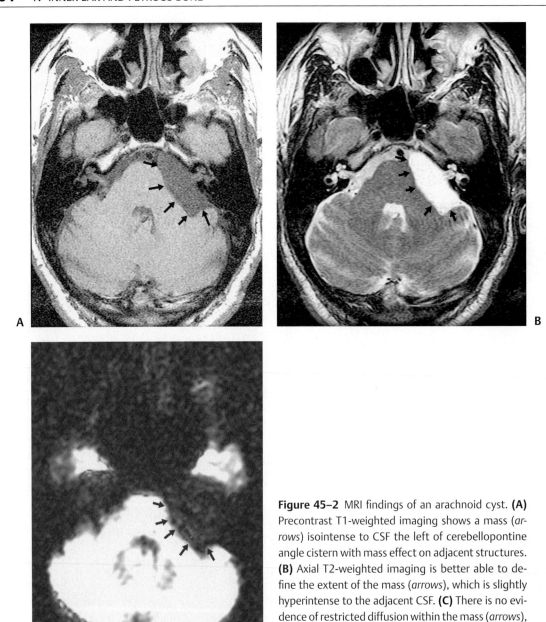

Figure 45–2 MRI findings of an arachnoid cyst. **(A)** Precontrast T1-weighted imaging shows a mass (*arrows*) isointense to CSF the left of cerebellopontine angle cistern with mass effect on adjacent structures. **(B)** Axial T2-weighted imaging is better able to define the extent of the mass (*arrows*), which is slightly hyperintense to the adjacent CSF. **(C)** There is no evidence of restricted diffusion within the mass (*arrows*), helping to differentiate this from an epidermoid cyst.

IMAGING PEARLS

- FLAIR and DWI MRI sequences are diagnostic in differentiating from arachnoid cyst. Epidermoids typically have increased DWI and FLAIR signal as compared with arachnoid cysts, which typically have low signal on DWI and FLAIR sequences.
- Other cystic lesions of the inner ear:
  ○ Arachnoid cyst: This cyst has mass effect on adjacent structures. It has CSF signal characteristics on all sequences, with no restricted diffusion and complete attenuation on FLAIR sequences.
  ○ Cystic meningioma and schwannoma: Both of these benign tumors show some degree of post-gadolinium enhancement on T1-weighted images.
  ○ Ependymoma: This may be predominantly cystic but is predominantly centered in the brainstem. Some enhancement is seen on MRI on gadolinium-enhanced scans.

○ Astrocytoma: This may be predominantly cystic. It arises from the fourth ventricle and may pedunculate in the CPA-IAC region. Some degree of enhancement is identified on gadolinium-enhanced MRI.

○ Cysticercus cyst: This may be considered in the endemic areas.

Suggested Readings

Altschuler EM, Jungries CA, Sekhar LN. Operative treatment of intracranial epidermoid cysts and cholesterol granulomas: Report of 21 cases. Neurosurgery 1990;26:606–614

Bonneville F, Sarrazin J-L, Marsot-Dupuch K. Unusual lesions of the cerebellopontine angle: a segmental approach. Radiographics 2001;21:419–438

Brackmann DE, Bartels LJ. Rare tumors of the cerebellopontine angle. Otolaryngol Head Neck Surg 1980;88:555–559

Dutt SN, Mirza S, Chavda SV. Radiologic differentiation of intracranial epidermoids from arachnoid cysts. Otol Neurotol 2002;23:84–92

Link MJ, Cohen PL, Breneman JC. Malignant squamous degeneration of a cerebellopontine angle epidermoid tumor: case report. J Neurosurg 2002;97:1237–1243

Pampliega-Pérez A, Martin-Estefania C, Caballe-Tura M. Aseptic meningitis caused by the rupture of an epidermoid cyst. Rev Neurol 2003;37:221–224

Singh S, Gibikote SV, Bannur U. Cysticercosis of the cerebellopontine angle cistern mimicking epidermoid inclusion cyst. Acta Neurol Scand 1999;99:260–263

Smirniotopoulos JG, Chiechi MV. Teratomas, dermoids, and epidermoids of the head and neck. Radiographics 1995;15:1437–1455

Tekkok IH, Cataltepe O, Saglam S. Dense epidermoid cyst of the cerebellopontine angle. Neuroradiology 1991;33:255–257

Yamakawa K, Shitara N, Genka S, et al. Clinical course and surgical prognosis of 33 cases of intracranial epidermoid tumors. Neurosurgery 1989;24:568–573

Zamzuri I, Abdullah J, Madhavan M, et al. A rare case of bleeding in a cerebellopontine angle epidermoid cyst. Med J Malaysia 2002;57:114–117

CHAPTER 46 Endolymphatic Sac Tumor

Vaishali Phalke

Epidemiology

This is a slow-growing tumor that arises from cells lining the endolymphatic sac. Most of the endolymphatic sac tumors (ELSTs) are sporadic. There is an association of ELST and von Hippel–Lindau (VHL) syndrome with the incidence of ELST, documented by magnetic resonance imaging (MRI), of 11% in patients with VHL. Patients with bilateral tumors are presumed to have VHL disease.

Clinical Features

Almost all patients present with hearing loss. Patients may also have symptoms of facial nerve palsy (60%), pulsatile tinnitus (50%), or even vertigo (20%).

Pathology

Macroscopically the tumors are reddish blue. These slow-growing tumors arising from the lining of the endolymphatic sac have a variable histopathologic appearance. Complex interdigitating papillary processes infiltrate surrounding connective tissue and bone. The papillary processes are generally embedded in sheets of dense fibrous tissue with recent and previous hemorrhage, cholesterol clefts, and scattered inflammatory cells. The papillary processes are lined with a single layer of low columnar to cuboidal epithelial cells resembling cells lining the endolymphatic sac. The cells have a small centrally placed ovoid nuclus with deeply eosinophilic homogeneous cytoplasm. There is no nuclear pleomorphism, and mitotic figures are absent. Tumor infiltration forms residual bone fragments that are seen as intratumoral calcifications on CT.

Treatment

The treatment of choice is complete surgical resection. There is no current role for radiation therapy or chemotherapy.

Imaging Findings

CT

Computed tomography (CT) demonstrates soft tissue mass that has aggressive characteristics and erodes the posterior wall of the temporal bone in the retrolabyrinthine region. The posterior margin of the tumor may have some thin rim of calcification with central spiculated calcifications seen in almost all cases within the tumor matrix.

When the tumors are large, they may extend into the cerebellopontine angle cistern, anteriorly into the cavernous sinus, or inferiorly to the skull base in the vicinity of the jugular foramen (**Fig. 46–1A**).

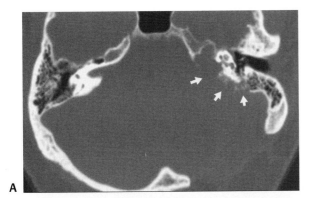

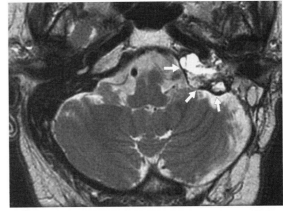

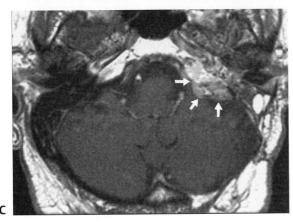

Figure 46–1 Computed tomography (CT) and magnetic resonance imaging (MRI) findings of an endolymphatic sac tumor. **(A)** High-resolution CT of the temporal bone shows erosion of the retrolabyrinthine temporal bone (*white arrows*) with some central spiculated calcifications. **(B)** MRI in the same patient shows the lesion (*arrows*) to have a heterogeneous appearance on T2-weighted images likely due to the presence of blood products. **(C)** Contrast-enhanced T1-weighted imaging shows heterogeneous enhancement within the lesion (*arrows*).

MRI

The appearance of the tumor on magnetic resonance imaging (MRI) varies with the size of the tumor. On the noncontrast T1-weighted scans, foci of high signal due to blood may be visualized. These foci are seen within the tumor matrix when they are larger than 3 cm and along the margin when smaller than 3 cm. When the tumors are larger than 2 cm, there may be flow voids seen within the tumor. On contrast-enhanced T1-weighted scans the tumor generally shows heterogeneous enhancement (**Fig. 46–1B,C**).

Angiography

The vascularity of the tumor varies with its size. Tumors less than 3 cm are supplied by branches of the external carotid artery, including the ascending pharyngeal, stylomastoid, and petrosal branch of the middle meningeal arteries. When the tumors are 3 cm or larger, they may be supplied by branches of the internal carotid artery and posterior circulation besides the branches of the external carotid artery. All tumors show hypervascular tumor blush.

IMAGING PEARLS _____

- CT and contrast-enhanced MRI are helpful to fully work up these tumors, especially when they are large.
- MR angiography and MR venography help in defining the vascular relationships.
- It is necessary to differentiate these tumors from metastasis from papillary thyroid carcinoma and renal cell carcinoma. Metastases are more destructive with no internal high-signal foci on precontrast T1-weighted imaging. Metastases also generally do not have a posterior rim of calcification on CT.
- The tumors may involve the skull base only when they are large and in the region of the jugular foramen when large. In those cases they would need to be differentiated from glomus jugulare and jugulotympanicum tumors, which characteristically erode the jugular foramen.

Suggested Readings

Gaffey MJ, Mills SE, Fechner RE. Aggressive papillary middle ear tumor. Am J Surg Pathol 1988;12:790–797

Heffner DK. Low grade adenocarcinoma of probable endolymphatic sac origin: a clinicopathologic study of 20 cases. Cancer 1989;64:2292–2302

Lo WW, Applegate LJ, Carberry JN. Endolymphatic sac tumors: Radiologic appearance. Radiology 1993;189:199–204

Manski TJ, Heffner DK, Glenn GM. Endolymphatic sac tumors. A source of morbid hearing loss in von-hippel-Lindau disease. JAMA 1997;277:1461–1466

Mukherji SK, Albernaz VS, Lo WW. Papillary endolymphatic sac tumors: CT, MR imaging and angiographic findings in 20 patients. Radiology 1997;202:801–808

Poe DS, Tarlov EC, Thomas CB. Aggressive papillary tumours of the temporal bone. Otolaryngol Head Neck Surg 1993;108:80–86

Richard S, David P, Marsot-Dupuch K. Central nervous system hemangioblastomas, endolymphatic sac tumors and Von Hippel Lindau disease. Neurosurg Rev 2000;23:1–22

CHAPTER 47 Transverse Temporal Bone Fractures
Diana Gomez-Hassan

Epidemiology

Transverse fractures are much less common than longitudinal fractures. Longitudinal fractures comprise 70 to 90% of temporal bone fractures, whereas transverse fractures account for approximately 10 to 30%. Specifically, these transverse fractures run perpendicular to the long axis of the petrous temporal bone. In reality, the majority of fractures run oblique to the axis of the petrous bone, and many abnormalities are associated with both types of temporal bone fractures. Transverse fractures usually occur as a result of blunt trauma to the occiput.

Clinical Features

Sensorineural hearing loss and vertigo occur more frequently with transverse fractures of the temporal bones. Sensorineural hearing loss occurs as a result of injury to the osseous labyrinth and cochlear and vestibular structures. In contrast to longitudinal fractures, conductive hearing loss occurs much less frequently because the ossicular chain is often spared. Vertigo can occur due to direct injury to the vestibular nerves or structures, but can also occur as a result of a perilymphatic fistula. Another clinical manifestation of transverse temporal bone fractures is immediate and complete facial paralysis. Delayed manifestations of temporal bone fractures include cerebrospinal fluid (CSF) otorrhea and meningitis.

Pathology

Transverse fractures typically result from trauma to the occiput or cranial-cervical junction. The line of force runs roughly anterior to posterior beginning near the jugular foramen or foramen magnum and extending toward the middle cranial fossa. When the fracture passes through the vestibulocochlear apparatus, both sensorineural hearing loss and disorders of equilibrium may occur. Injury to the facial nerve is common in this type of injury as well, because the fracture often courses close to the labyrinthine segment of the facial nerve. The fracture line can extend into the internal auditory canal. The fracture may also involve the tegmen tympani and tegmen mastoideum. As a result, patients are at risk for CSF leaks and meningitis.

Treatment

Early treatment is directed toward repair of CSF otorrhea. This can occur by conservative management, which may include bed rest with the head elevated by 15 to 25 degrees, avoidance of straining, and antibiotic therapy to prevent meningitis. More aggressive therapy includes placement of a lumbar drain or even surgical patch repair.

Treatment is also directed toward prevention of facial nerve paralysis, especially in cases when the paralysis is immediate in onset and complete after the trauma. Operative intervention is often necessary in reversing or at least limiting the degree of nerve impingement.

Damage to the cochlear and vestibular structures can result in profound sensorineural hearing loss and vertigo. The vertigo may resolve with time (3 to 6 months) due to compensation, but the sensorineural hearing loss may require cochlear implantation.

Imaging Findings

CT

High-resolution bone algorithm shows a perpendicular fracture line relative to the long axis of the petrous temporal bone. The fracture line may extend through the semicircular canal, vestibule, or cochlea. The course of the fracture line may also extend into segments of the facial nerve. The most commonly involved portions are the labyrinthine, anterior genu, and tympanic segments of the facial nerve (**Fig. 47–1, Fig. 47–2,** and **Fig. 47–3**).

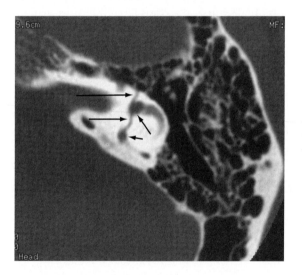

Figure 47–1 Axial computed tomography (CT) demonstrates a transverse fracture of the petrous portion of the temporal bone. The fracture line (*large arrows*) courses through the crus (*small arrows*) of the semicircular canals.

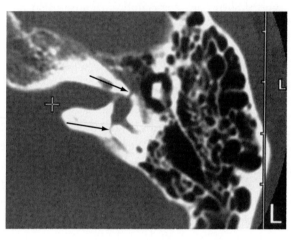

Figure 47–2 Axial image illustrates a transverse fracture that extends through the vestibule toward the tympanic segment of the facial nerve.

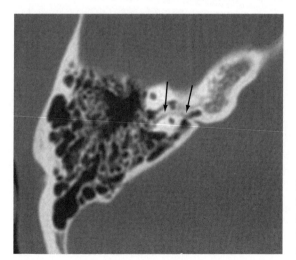

Figure 47–3 Axial CT obtained through the left petrous apex shows a curvilinear lucency (*arrows*). This is the normal appearance of the canal of the arcuate artery and is not a transverse fracture; hence the term *pseudofracture*.
(Courtesy of Michael Gordon, MD, PhD.)

MRI

Magnetic resonance imaging (MRI) has poor specificity in identifying temporal bone fractures. It may be helpful in identifying associated temporal contusion.

IMAGING PEARLS

- The fracture line extends along a perpendicular axis to the petrous temporal bone.
- Sensorineural hearing loss occurs more frequently with these fractures.
- Although much less frequent than longitudinal fractures, these fractures occur as a result of blunt trauma to the occiput.
- The groove for the arcuate artery courses perpendicular along the petrous apex. This is a normal variant and should not be confused with a transverse fracture.

Suggested Readings

Cannon CR, Jahrsdoerfer RA. Temporal bone fractures. Review of 90 cases. Arch Otolaryngol 1983;109:285–288

Freeman J. Temporal bone fractures and cholesteatoma. Ann Otol Rhinol Laryngol 1983;92:558–560

Swartz JD, Curtin HD. Temporal bone trauma. In: Som PM, Curtin HD, eds. Head and Neck Imaging, 4th ed. St. Louis: Mosby, 2003:1230–1244

CHAPTER 48 Longitudinal Temporal Bone Fractures

Diana Gomez-Hassan

Epidemiology

Longitudinal temporal bone fractures are often the result of blunt head trauma to the temporal or parietal bone with the force transmitted from lateral to medial. Specifically, these fractures occur along the long axis of the petrous temporal bone. Although most fractures of the temporal bone can be complex, longitudinal fractures are more common (70 to 90%) than transverse fractures (10 to 30%).

Clinical Features

Many patients with acute temporal bone fractures present with hemotympanum, hearing loss, or, less commonly, vertigo. Lack of resolution of conductive hearing loss often is due to ossicular chain discontinuity. Longitudinal fractures can also be directly associated with facial nerve paralysis if there is involvement of the internal auditory canal, but these symptoms can often be delayed and incomplete. This often occurs as a result of displaced fragments within the middle ear.

Pathology

Patients with longitudinal fractures are at increased risk of developing cholesteatoma secondary to deposition of squamous epithelial debris into the middle ear along the fracture line. The fracture may involve the tegmen tympani and tegmen mastoideum. As a result, patients are at risk for cerebrospinal fluid (CSF) leaks and meningitis.

Treatment

Longitudinal fractures can result in conductive hearing loss, which may resolve with time if the ossicular chain is not disrupted. However, disruption or damage to the ossicular chain may require surgical intervention and ossicular bone reconstruction.

As with transverse fractures, treatment of longitudinal fractures may also be directed toward repair of CSF otorrhea. This can occur by conservative management, which may include bed rest with the head elevated by 15 to 25 degrees, avoidance of straining, and antibiotic therapy to prevent meningitis. More aggressive therapy includes placement of a lumbar drain or even surgical patch repair.

Treatment is also directed toward prevention of facial nerve paralysis, especially in cases when the paralysis is complete and immediate in onset after the trauma. Operative intervention is often necessary in reversing or at least limiting the degree of nerve impingement.

Imaging Findings

CT

A linear lucency is typically seen coursing through the temporal bone along the long axis of the petrous pyramid of the temporal bone, best viewed on an axial high-resolution thin-section (1 to 1.25 mm in thickness) computed tomography (CT). The fracture line is also accompanied with opacification of the

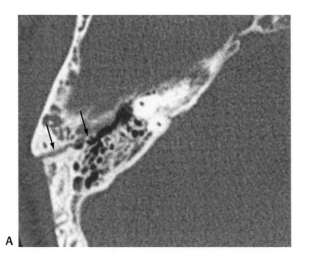

A

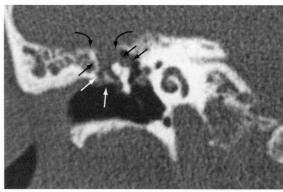

B

Figure 48–1 (A) Axial computed tomography (CT) through the temporal bone demonstrates a linear longitudinal fracture (*arrows*) extending through the petrous bone and mastoid air cell. The mucosal thickening in the mastoid air cell is likely due to posttraumatic hemorrhage. **(B)** Coronal image obtained in the same patient shows a fracture of the tegmen tympani (*curved arrow*) associated with a soft tissue abnormality (*straight arrows*). The soft tissue abnormality was due to an encephalocele that was extending through the posttraumatic defect.

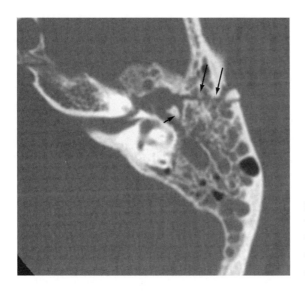

Figure 48–2 Axial CT demonstrates a longitudinal fracture through the left temporal bone (*long arrows*). Images through the middle ear cavity show ossicular disruption of the incudomalleolar joint. The short process of the incus is seen (*small arrow*), but the malleolus has been dislocated.

mastoid air cells and middle ear cavity secondary to either hemorrhage or CSF otorrhea. Laterally, the fracture frequently involves the external auditory canal. Medially, the fracture line courses lateral to the carotid canal near the foramen spinosum. Longitudinal fractures are associated with ossicular disruption often at the incudomalleolar joint (**Fig. 48–1** and **Fig. 48–2**).

MRI

Magnetic resonance imaging (MRI) has poor specificity in identifying temporal bone fractures. It may be helpful in identifying associated temporal contusion.

IMAGING PEARLS

- The fracture line extends parallel to the petrous pyramid of the temporal bone.
- This fracture occurs more frequently than transverse fractures.
- Conductive hearing loss due to ossicular disruption more commonly occurs with these fractures.

Suggested Readings

Cannon CR, Jahrsdoerfer RA. Temporal bone fractures. Review of 90 cases. Arch Otolaryngol 1983;109:285–288

Freeman J. Temporal bone fractures and cholesteatoma. Ann Otol Rhinol Laryngol 1983;92:558–560

Swartz JD, Curtin HD. Temporal bone trauma. In: Som PM, Curtin HD, eds. Head and Neck Imaging, 4th ed. St. Louis: Mosby 2003:1230–1244

CHAPTER 49 Mastoidectomy

Ellen G. Hoeffner

Epidemiology

Mastoidectomy is performed for suppurative disease of the middle ear and mastoid; cochlear implantation; access to the cerebellopontine angle, skull base, and petrous apex; labyrinthectomy; endolymphatic sac decompression; repair of facial nerve disorders; and cerebrospinal fluid leaks.

Clinical Features

A variety of mastoidectomy procedures can be performed, including simple, canal wall up (closed cavity or intact canal wall), canal wall down (open cavity), modified radical, and radical mastoidectomies. This chapter focuses on canal wall up and canal wall down mastoidectomies in the setting of chronic otitis media and cholesteatoma.

No prospective, randomized trials have been performed to indicate whether the canal wall up or canal wall down mastoidectomy is the definitive procedure for the treatment of cholesteatoma. Both procedures have been used successfully to treat cholesteatoma. The canal wall down approach has a lower incidence of residual or recurrent disease and can eradicate disease and preserve or restore hearing in a single operative procedure. It may also provide better intraoperative visualization of middle ear structures. However, the disadvantage of the canal wall down approach is generally a longer time for healing postoperatively and possible long-term local care of the mastoid cavity.

With the canal wall up approach, the normal anatomy is preserved, healing is quicker, and there is generally less need for long-term care of the operative site. The disadvantage of this technique is poorer operative exposure of disease extent, resulting in the need for greater surgical manipulation, longer operative time, and a higher incidence of residual or recurrent disease that may require further operative treatment.

Treatment

In a simple mastoidectomy, there is limited removal of mastoid air cells without entering the epitympanum or mastoid antrum. The ossicles cannot be directly visualized.

With the canal wall up mastoidectomy, there is resection of all mastoid air cells, the overlying cortex, and Körner septum with preservation of the posterior and superior walls of the external auditory canal (EAC). The resulting surgically created cavity, termed the "mastoid bowl," communicates with the antrum and epitympanum, allowing direct visualization of the ossicles.

Canal wall down procedures can be subdivided into modified radical and radical mastoidectomies. For both of these procedures, the posterior superior wall of the EAC is removed along with the mastoid air cells, such that the EAC communicates with the mastoid cavity. A radical mastoidectomy also involves the removal of the malleus and incus while preserving the stapes superstructure. With a modified radical mastoidectomy, the entire ossicular chain is preserved or reconstructed.

Imaging Findings

CT

Computed tomography (CT) is the imaging modality of choice in assessing the air spaces and osseous structures of the postoperative mastoid. Specific imaging features allow the radiologist to distinguish a canal wall up from a canal wall down procedure on CT. In a canal wall up procedure the posterior and superior wall of the EAC is preserved and is visible on CT images. The mastoid bowl communicates with the antrum and epitympanum. Imaging after a canal wall down procedure reveals absence of the posterior and superior wall of the EAC. Additional findings depend on the reason for the mastoidectomy and any additional surgery. For example, ossicular prostheses may be present if the native ossicles were diseased. The posterior wall of the IAC may be resected with or without resection of the semicircular canals, if access to the seventh and eighth cranial nerves is necessary.

Normally, following a mastoidectomy there should be no soft tissue within the mastoid bowl or tympanic cavity. Some patients (estimated to be approximately 20%) imaged after a mastoidectomy have nonspecific soft tissue within the tympanomastoid cavity. This soft tissue may consist of inflammatory hyperplastic mucosa, granulation tissue, fluid, cholesterol granuloma, or cholesteatoma. CT generally cannot distinguish among these possibilities. A cholesteatoma may be suggested if there is an epitympanic soft tissue mass with focal bony destruction (**Fig. 49–1, Fig. 49–2,** and **Fig. 49–3**)

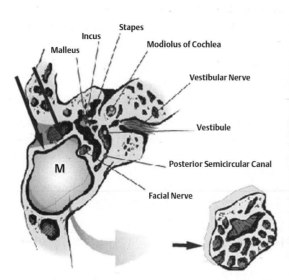

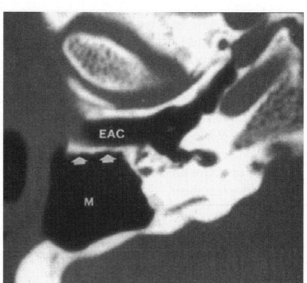

A

B

Figure 49–1 Canal wall up mastoidectomy. **(A)** Diagram demonstrates the mastoid bowl (M), the intact posterior wall of the external auditory canal (EAC) (*long arrows*), and resected mastoid air cells (*short arrow*). (See Color Plate 49–1A) **(B)** Axial computed tomography (CT) shows an air-filled mastoid bowl (M) with an intact posterior wall of the external auditory canal (EAC) (*arrows*).

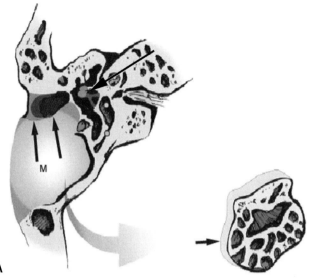

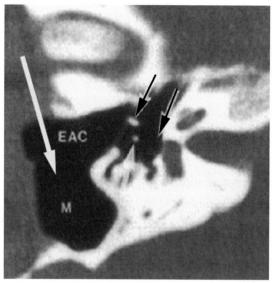

Figure 49–2 Canal wall down mastoidectomy with ossicular preservation. **(A)** Diagram demonstrates the mastoid bowl (M), the resection of the posterior wall of the EAC (*medium black arrows*), and resected mastoid air cells (*short black arrow*). The ossicles have been preserved (*longest black arrow*).

(See Color Plate 49–2A) **(B)** Axial CT shows resection of the posterior wall of the EAC (*long arrow*), such that the EAC communicates with the mastoid bowl (M). The ossicles have been preserved (*short arrows*).

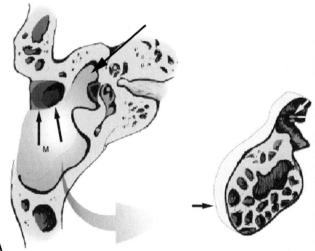

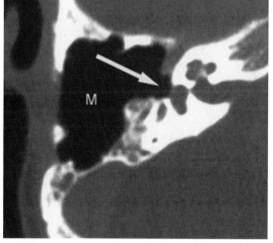

Figure 49–3 Canal wall down mastoidectomy with ossicular resection. **(A)** Diagram demonstrates the mastoid bowl (M) and the resection of the posterior wall of the EAC (*long black arrows*). The ossicles (*white arrow*) have been resected along

with the mastoid air cells (*short black arrow*). (See Color Plate 49–3A) **(B)** Axial CT shows resection of the posterior wall of the EAC, such that the EAC communicates with the mastoid bowl (M). The ossicles have been resected (*arrow*).

MRI

Magnetic resonance imaging (MRI) is generally reserved for assessing neural elements, the membranous labyrinth and fluid, or soft tissue–filled cavities of the temporal bone in the postmastoidectomy patient. Recurrent cholesteatomas appear hyperintense on diffusion-weighted MRI and do not enhance, except for around their periphery. Homogeneous enhancement is present on delayed, postcontrast images of granulation tissue.

IMAGING PEARLS _____

- CT is the main imaging modality used to assess bone and air spaces of the postoperative mastoid and allows the radiologist to determine the type of procedure performed.
- The posterior and superior walls of the EAC are preserved in a canal wall up mastoidectomy and are absent in patients who have had canal wall down procedures.
- Normally the mastoid bowl and tympanic cavity is free of any soft tissue opacification. If soft tissue is present, MRI may be helpful in determining its etiology.

Suggested Readings

Hulka GF, McElveen JT. A randomized, blinded study of canal wall up verses canal wall down mastoidectomy determining the differences in viewing middle ear anatomy and pathology. Am J Otol 1998;19:574–578

Kosling S, Bootz F. CT and MR imaging after middle ear surgery. Eur J Radiol 2001;40:113–118

Lambert PR. Mastoidectomy. In: Cummings CW, Flint PW, Harker LA, et al. Otolaryngology: Head and Neck Surgery, 4th ed. Philadelphia: Elsevier Mosby, 2005:3075–3086

Mukherji SK, Mancuso AA, Kotzur IM. CT of the temporal bone: findings after mastoidectomy, ossicular reconstruction, and cochlear implantation. AJR Am J Roentgenol 1994;163:1467–1471

Nemzek WR, Swartz JD. Temporal bone: inflammatory disease. In: Som PM, Curtin HD, eds. Head and Neck Imaging, 4th ed. St. Louis: Mosby, 2003:1173–1229

Williams MT, Ayache D. Imaging of the postoperative middle ear. Eur Radiol 2004;14:482–495

CHAPTER 50 Ossicular Replacement Prostheses
Ellen G. Hoeffner

Epidemiology

Synthetic ossicular protheses are commonly indicated in patients with ossicular disruption or destruction caused by chronic otitis media and cholesteatoma. They may also be used in patients with congenital ossicular malformations, posttraumatic injuries, and otosclerosis. The prosthesis is used to restore the integrity of the ossicular chain and allow sound waves to be transmitted to the inner ear.

Clinical Features

The type of synthetic ossicular prosthesis used is generally determined by the extent of ossicular damage or disease, the properties of the device, and the surgeon's preference. In disease limited to the oval window, a stapedectomy or stapedotomy is usually performed and the stapes superstructure (head, neck, and anterior and posterior crura) replaced by a prosthesis. For incudostapedial joint disease, a synthetic prosthesis or autologous bone may be used. A partial ossicular replacement prosthesis (PORP) or total ossicular replacement prosthesis (TORP) is employed when more extensive ossicular reconstruction is necessary. Although the terms PORP and TORP are registered trademarks, they are commonly used to refer to two basic prosthetic configurations used to reconstruct the ossicular chain. The term PORP is commonly used when the stapes is intact and mobile, whereas the term TORP is used when the superstructure of the stapes is absent, but the footplate is present and mobile.

Malfunction of ossicular prostheses can occur and should be clinically suspected when there is an increase in conductive hearing loss. Malfunction can be the result of recurrent middle ear disease (otitis media or cholesteatoma), granulation tissue or adhesions, or displacement (subluxation, dislocation, or extrusion) of the prosthesis.

Treatment

Otosclerosis and congenital abnormalities are the most common indications for stapes reconstruction with prosthesis placement. Other indications include posttraumatic injuries, adhesions, and tympanosclerosis. In a stapedectomy, the stapes superstructure and part or all of the footplate are resected to open the oval window and allow sound to enter the labyrinth. A wire or piston prosthesis is used to reconstruct a conductive bridge between the incus and labyrinth. A stapedotomy is a newer procedure in which the stapes superstructure is resected, but the footplate preserved. A small hole is drilled in the footplate, and a wire piston is advanced through this small opening. Studies comparing the two procedures have revealed slightly better early and late postoperative air-conduction thresholds and a lower rate of postoperative sensorineural hearing loss in patients undergoing a stapedotomy. Vertigo and reparative granuloma formation are also less frequent with stapedotomy. Complications related to the stapes prosthesis include displacement, migration, or extrusion; resorption of the long process of the incus by direct pressure or foreign-body reaction; fracture or bending of prosthesis; vestibular perforation, often in the setting of increased negative middle ear pressure caused by eustachian tube dysfunction; perilymphatic fistula; post-stapedectomy granuloma; and fibrosis.

The incus is the most vulnerable ossicle with regard to traumatic and infectious injury. Damage to the incus can occur with an intact malleus handle and stapes. Three main types of incus prostheses—homograft, autograft, or allograft—may be used in this setting. Usually, an incus interposition procedure is performed, in which the native incus is removed, sculpted to a suitable size and shape, and interposed between the malleus and stapes. Potential complications of incus interposition include displacement, absorption, and harboring microorganisms. Alternatively, a homologous ossicle or synthetic prosthesis may be used. With homologous ossicular prostheses there is the risk of transmitting disease such as HIV, hepatitis, or Creutzfeldt-Jakob disease and the need to store and reconstitute the prosthesis. Subluxation, incudal necrosis, granuloma formation, recurrent cholesteatoma, and ankylosis are potential complications of incus interposition.

Synthetic prostheses are now the most commonly used and are available in two basic tack-like configurations: a PORP and a TORP. A PORP extends from the medial surface of the tympanic membrane or occasionally the malleus to the head of the stapes, whereas a TORP extends from the tympanic membrane or malleus to the stapes footplate or oval window. Synthetic prostheses are generally a composite, with the head made of hydroxyapatite, a biocompatible material that can bond to tissue, but is difficult to sculpt and modify. The shaft of the prosthesis may be made of Plasti-Pore (Medtronic Xiomed, Minneapolis, Minnesota), a high-density polyethylene sponge product, a fluoroplastic or a polymer of hydroxyapatite and polyethylene, all of which can be easily cut to the appropriate length. The specific shape of the prostheses varies among manufacturers. More recently titanium ossicular prostheses were introduced, their use first being reported in 1999. They also come in a TORP and PORP configuration.

Postoperative complications following placement of TORP or PORP include subluxation and extrusion. Encasement of the prosthesis by granulation tissue or recurrent cholesteatoma may result in subluxation. Extrusion of the prosthesis occurs most commonly with allografts that directly abut the tympanic membrane. The incidence of extrusion is less if a cartilage graft is placed between the tympanic membrane and the prosthesis or if the prosthesis abuts the undersurface of the manubrium, rather than the tympanic membrane directly.

Imaging Findings

CT

Once ossicular prostheses are implanted, computed tomography (CT) is the main imaging modality used to assess the position of the prosthesis and evaluate any complications. Regardless of composition, ossicular prostheses appear as radiodensities on CT. The various proprietary protheses have a characteristic configuration that can be identified on CT. Postoperative imaging is usually obtained in patients who present with new conductive hearing loss, in which case CT is useful in identifying the cause.

Stapes Prosthesis

In general, a stapes prothesis should extend from the lenticular process of the incus to the oval window. Dislocation or subluxation of the prosthesis is the most common repairable cause of stapes prosthetic failure. The medial end of the prosthesis is most often displaced inferior and posterior to the oval window, whereas the lateral aspect of the prosthesis can be displaced inferiorly from the long process of the incus. Such displacements are often the result of resorptive osteitis of the long process of the incus caused by direct pressure erosion by or foreign-body reaction in response to the prosthesis. In the extreme, the prosthesis may be extruded and identified within the dependent portion of the middle ear, outside of the tympanic cavity or be completely absent. The prosthesis can also fracture or bend.

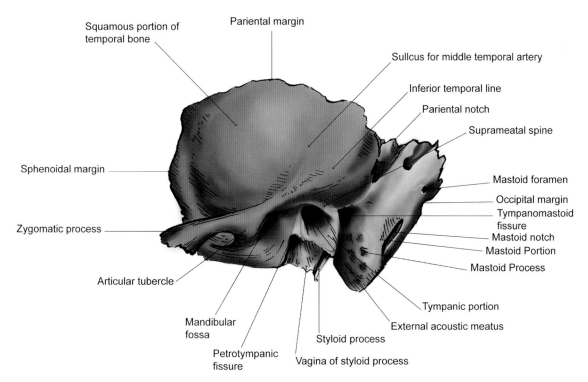

Color Plate 1–1A Labeled schematic illustrations of the lateral surface anatomy of the temporal bone. (See **Figure 1–1A**, page 2)

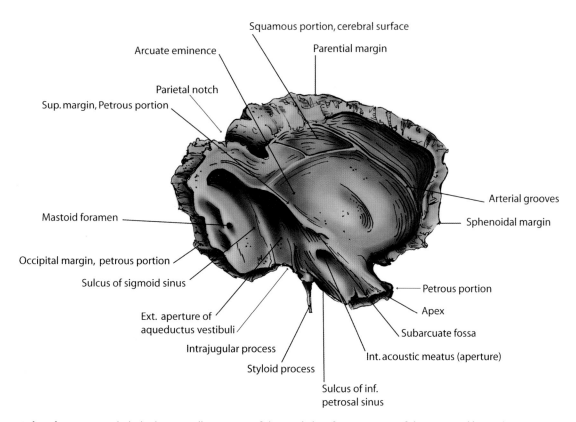

Color Plate 1–1B Labeled schematic illustrations of the medial surface anatomy of the temporal bone. (See **Figure 1–1B**, page 2)

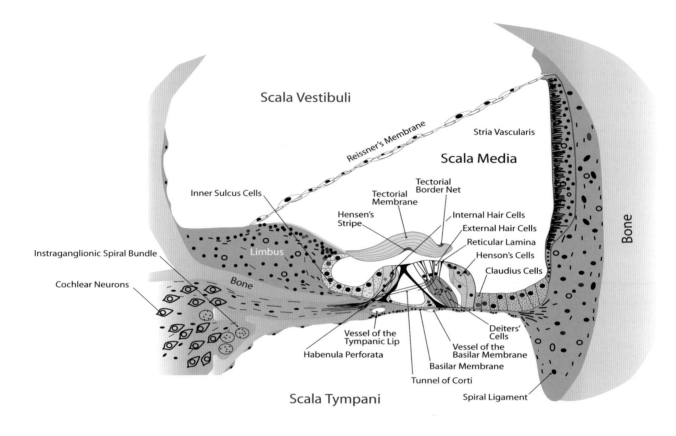

Color Plate 5–1 Schematic illustration of the anatomy of the cochlea and organ of Corti. (See **Figure 5–1**, page 20)

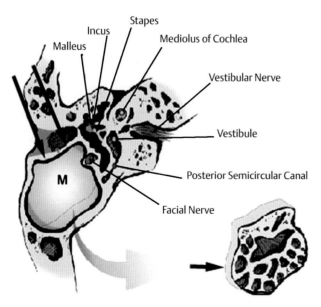

Color Plate 49–1A Canal wall up mastoidectomy. Diagram demonstrates the mastoid bowl (M), the intact posterior wall of the external auditory canal (EAC) (*long arrows*), and resected mastoid air cells (*short arrow*). (See **Figure 49–1A**, page 176)

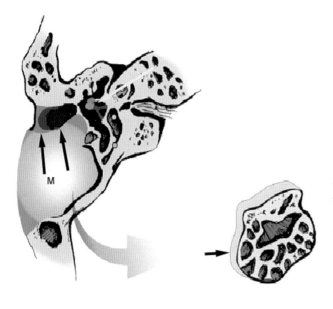

Color Plate 49–2A Canal wall down mastoidectomy with ossicular preservation. Diagram demonstrates the mastoid bowl (M), the resection of the posterior wall of the EAC (*medium black arrows*), and resected mastoid air cells (*short black arrow*). The ossicles have been preserved (*longest black arrow*). (See **Figure 49–2A**, page 177)

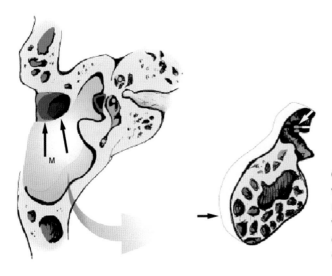

Color Plate 49–3A Canal wall down mastoidectomy with ossicular resection. Diagram demonstrates the mastoid bowl (M) and the resection of the posterior wall of the EAC (*long black arrows*). The ossicles (*white arrow*) have been resected along with the mastoid air cells (*short black arrow*). (See **Figure 49–3A**, page 177)

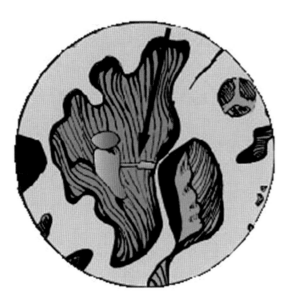

Color Plate 50–1A Stapes prosthesis. Diagram indicating stapes prosthesis (*arrow*) extending from incus to oval window. (See **Figure 50–1A**, page 181)

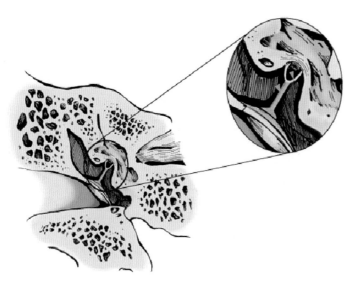

Color Plate 50–3A Partial ossicular replacement prosthesis (PORP). Diagram shows the PORP (*blue arrowhead*) extending medially from the tympanic membrane to articulate with the head of the stapes (*orange arrowhead*). (See **Figure 50–3A**, page 183)

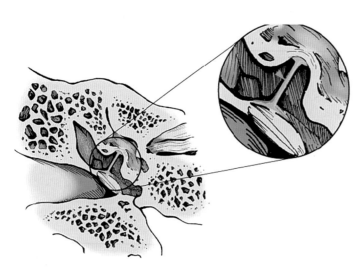

Color Plate 50–4A Total ossicular replacement prosthesis (TORP). Diagram of a TORP (*blue arrowhead*) extending from the tympanic membrane to the oval window. (See **Figure 50–4A**, page 183)

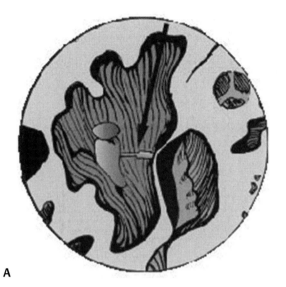

A

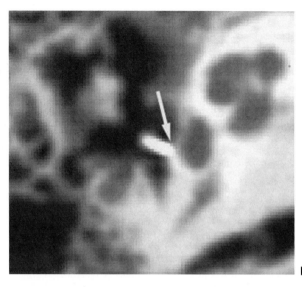

B

Figure 50–1 Stapes prosthesis. **(A)** Diagram indicating stapes prosthesis (*arrow*) extending from incus to oval window. (See Color Plate 50–1A) **(B)** Axial computed tomog-raphy (CT) image showing articulation of stapes prosthesis with oval window (*arrow*). The articulation with the lenticu-lar process of the incus is out of the image plane.

In patients presenting with vertigo, tinnitus, dysequilibrium, or sensorineural hearing loss, CT should be obtained to look for vestibular perforation or perilymphatic fistula. Increased negative middle ear pressure can force the prosthesis into the vestibule. This is easily visualized on CT, with the medial end of the prosthesis extending through the oval window into the vestibule and an air gap between the lateral end of the prosthesis and the incus. A perilymphatic fistula may be suggested by the presence of pneumolabyrinth or a new, unexplained middle ear effusion.

Normally, no soft tissue is present in the oval window niche 4 to 6 weeks after placement of the prosthesis. If soft tissue is seen beyond this time frame, granuloma or fibrosis should be considered.

Other abnormalities to assess on CT include bone overgrowth at the oval window, due to progressive otosclerosis or bone repair following excessive drilling at surgery, and obliteration of the oval window by otosclerosis (**Fig. 50–1**).

Incus Interposition

In this procedure the short process of the homograft incus points laterally and is situated beneath the manubrium of the malleus. The long process projects medially and is placed on the head of the stapes or the stapedial footplate if the superstructure is absent or resected. Complications detectable on CT include subluxation, incudal necrosis, reparative granuloma formation, and recurrent cholesteatoma. Progressive soft tissue opacification of the middle ear with ossicle erosion suggests recurrent cholest-eatoma, whereas abnormal soft tissue only suggests granuloma (**Fig. 50–2**).

PORP and TORP

The configuration of most PORPs and TORPs is that of a head with a shaft. The shaft of a PORP is gener-ally shorter and thicker than that of a TORP. The head of the prosthesis is directed laterally, abutting the tympanic membrane or, less often, the malleus. The shaft projects medially and extends to the head of the stapes (PORP) or the stapes footplate/oval window (TORP). Subluxation of these prostheses most often occurs at the articulation with the stapes or oval window. An air gap between the prosthesis and

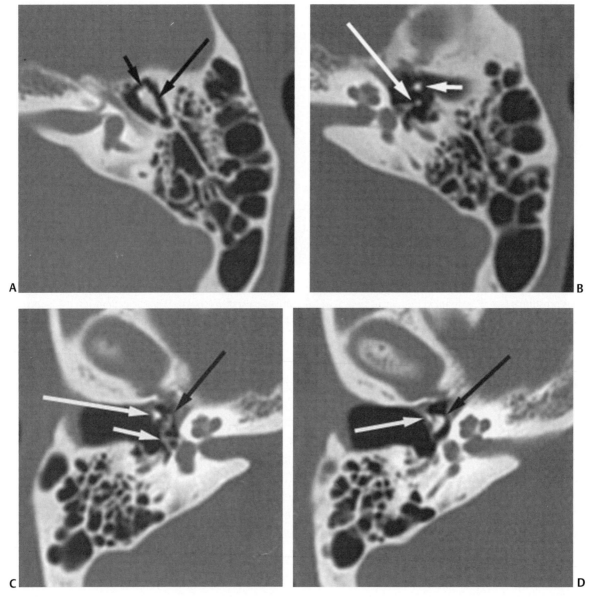

Figure 50–2 Incus interposition. **(A)** Axial CT image of the left ear showing normal articulation between the short process of the incus (*long arrow*) and the head of the malleus (*short arrow*). **(B)** Axial CT image slightly inferior to **A**, demonstrating normal articulation between the lenticular process of the incus and the head of the stapes (*long arrow*) and the manubrium of the malleus (*short arrow*). **(C)** Axial CT of the right ear in the same patient showing the incus (*black arrow*) rotated such that it is positioned between the head of the stapes medially (*short white arrow*) and the manubrium of the malleus laterally (*long white arrow*). **(D)** Axial CT image slightly inferior to **C** with interposed incus (*black arrow*) articulating with manubrium of malleus (*white arrow*).

the oval window suggests subluxation. Abnormal soft tissue encasing a prosthesis may be due to recurrent cholesteatoma or granulation tissue and can cause conductive hearing loss from dampening of the pistonlike action of the prosthesis during sound transmission. Recurrent cholesteatoma or granulation tissue can also lead to subluxation of the prosthesis (**Fig. 50–3** and **Fig. 50–4**).

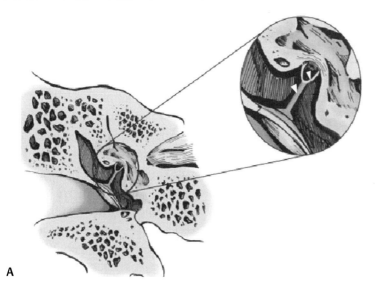

A

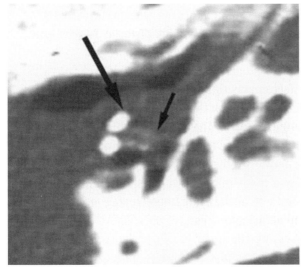

B

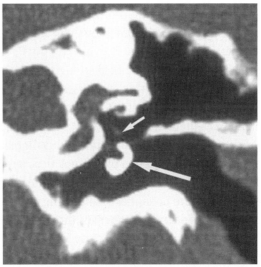

C

Figure 50–3 Partial ossicular replacement prosthesis (PORP). **(A)** Diagram shows the PORP (*upper right arrowhead*) extending medially from the tympanic membrane to articulate with the head of the stapes (*lower left arrowhead*). (See Color Plate 50–3A) **(B)** Axial CT image with PORP extending from tympanic membrane (*long arrow*) to head of stapes (*short arrow*) in a partially opacified middle ear. **(C)** Coronal CT image showing a subluxed PORP (*long arrow*) displaced inferiorly, away from the head of the stapes (*short arrow*).

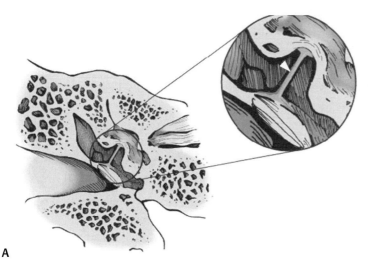

A

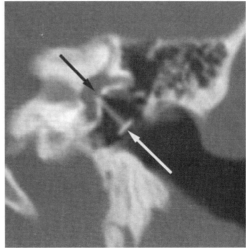

B

Figure 50–4 Total ossicular replacement prosthesis (TORP). **(A)** Diagram of a TORP (*arrowhead*) extending from the tympanic membrane to the oval window. (See Color Plate 50–4A) **(B)** Coronal CT image of a TORP extending from the tympanic membrane (*white arrow*) to the oval window (*black arrow*).

MRI

Magnetic resonance imaging (MRI) is infrequently indicated to assess the middle ear after placement of an ossicular prosthesis. The prostheses, regardless of composition, appear as a signal void on MRI, as does surrounding air and bone. Thus ossicular prostheses are not visible on MRI. Additionally, prostheses that contain metal generate susceptibility artifact, resulting in distortion of surrounding structures.

If a patient does require an MRI for postoperative assessment or for some other reason following placement of a middle ear prosthesis, the safety of imaging such a patient with an implant that may be ferromagnetic or rendered ferromagnetic by the manufacturing process is a primary concern. The concern is that the electromagnetic fields generated by MRI scanners may cause movement or heating of the prosthesis. Most ossicular prostheses have not displayed ferromagnetism when tested with a 1.5-tesla (T) static magnet, though there have been a few exceptions. One stapedectomy piston prosthesis made of ferromagnetic stainless steel was grossly displaced by the MRI scanner; this prosthesis was later recalled and patients who had the prosthesis implanted before the recall were given MRI safety warning cards. More recently, several stapes prostheses made of nonferromagnetic material showed gross movement when placed in a 1.5-T scanner. The authors of this study theorized that the manufacturing process induced the ferromagnetism and suggested testing every stapes prosthesis for movement, by placing the prosthesis in a sterile Petri dish and using a handheld sterile magnet, prior to implantation.

With the advent of higher field strength clinical magnets, studies performed on middle ear prostheses have shown that multiple prostheses made of nonferromagnetic stainless steel do show displacement when tested ex vivo at 3-T field strength or higher, even though these same prostheses may have shown no movement in MRI scanners of 1.5-T field strength or lower. The clinical significance of ex vivo movement of prostheses is uncertain; when implanted in cadaveric temporal bones or animal models, these prostheses remained in proper position, without demonstrable movement or damage to the oval window, even at field strengths of 3 T or higher. Prostheses made of metals such as titanium, platinum, nickel, or nitinol are presumably safe in the MRI environment, as these are nonferromagnetic and cannot acquire ferromagnetic properties through the manufacturing process.

Magnetic resonance imaging may be useful in assessing the inner ear in patients who develop labyrinthine symptoms, such as vertigo or sensorineural hearing loss, after placement of a prosthesis. MRI may detect labyrinthine hemorrhage in cases of intravestibular protrusion of a prosthesis, fibrous obliteration of the labyrinth, or spread of granulation tissue into the inner ear.

IMAGING PEARLS _____

- CT is the main imaging modality in evaluating patients with middle ear prostheses. CT can assess the position of the prosthesis and most complications.
- All prostheses appear as radiodensities on CT, regardless of composition. The most commonly used prostheses come in a PORP and TORP configuration.
- Subluxation or dislocation is one of the most common complications of ossicular prosthesis surgery. As such the radiologist should be aware of the normal position of the main types of prostheses and patterns of dislocation.
- Although MRI is safe in the majority of patients with ossicular prostheses, attention should be given to verifying the type of prosthesis present and its behavior in magnetic fields of varying strengths. The risk-benefit ratio should be considered before allowing patients with some prostheses to be scanned and discussed with patients as well as the other physicians involved in the patients' care.

Suggested Readings

Applebaum EL, Valvassori CE. Further studies on the effects of magnetic resonance fields on middle ear implants. Ann Otol Rhinol Laryngol 1990;99:801–804

El-Kashlan HK, Harker LA. Tympanoplasty and ossiculoplasty. In: Cummings CW, Flint PW, Harker LA, et al. Otolaryngology: Head and Neck Surgery, 4th ed. Philadelphia: Elsevier Mosby, 2005:3058–3074

Fritsch MH, Gutt JJ. Ferromagnetic movements of middle ear implants and stapes prostheses in a 3T magnetic resonance field. Otol Neurotol 2005;26:225–230

Hillman TA, Shelton C. Ossicular chain reconstruction: titanium verses Plastipore. Laryngoscope 2003;113:1731–1735

Hirsch BE, Weissman JL, Curtin HD. Imaging of ossicular prostheses. Otolaryngol Head Neck Surg 1994;111:494–496

Ho SY, Battista RA, Wiet RJ. Early results with titanium ossicular implants. Otol Neurotol 2003;24:149–152

Iurato S, Mariono G, Onofri M. Hearing results of ossiculoplasty in Austin-Kartush group A patients. Otol Neurotol 2001;22:140–144

Kosling S, Bootz F. CT and MR imaging after middle ear surgery. Eur J Radiol 2001;40:113–118

Mukherji SK, Castillo M. The posttherapeutic temporal bone. In: Jinkins JR, ed. Posttherapeutic neuro-diagnostic imaging. Philadelphia: Lippencott-Raven, 1997:89–102

Mukherji SK, Mancuso AA, Kotzur IM. CT of the temporal bone: findings after mastoidectomy, ossicular reconstruction, and cochlear implantation. AJR Am J Roentgenol 1994;163:1467–1471

O'Reilly RC, Cass SP, Hirsh BE. Ossiculoplasty using incus interposition: Hearing results and analysis of middle ear risk index. Otol Neurotol 2005;26:853–858

Shellock FG, Morisoli S, Kanal E. MR procedures and biomedical implants, materials and devices: 1993 update. Radiology 1993;189:587–599

Stone JA, Mukherji SK, Jewett BS. CT evaluation of prosthetic ossicular reconstruction procedures: what the otologist needs to know. Radiographics 2000;20:593–605

Stupp CH, Dalchow C, Grun D. Three years of experience with titanium implants in the middle ear. Laryngorhinootologie 1999;78:299–303

Syms MJ. Safety of magnetic resonance imaging of stapes prostheses. Laryngoscope 2005;115:381–390

Syms MJ, Peterman GW. Magnetic resonance imaging of stapes prostheses. Am J Otol 2000;21:494–498

Williams MD, Antonelli PJ, Williams LS. Middle ear prosthesis displacement in high-strength magnetic fields. Otol Neurotol 2001;22:158–161

Williams MT, Ayache D. Imaging of the postoperative middle ear. Eur Radiol 2004;14:482–495

CHAPTER 51 Cochlear Implantation

Ellen G. Hoeffner

Epidemiology

Cochlear implants (CIs) have become the accepted treatment in patients with severe to profound bilateral sensorineural hearing loss (SNHL) who receive little benefit from conventional hearing aids.

Clinical Features

For patients under consideration for a CI, a complete hearing history must be obtained, a neurotologic and head and neck examination must be performed, and a series of hearing tests must be administered. Certain levels of hearing loss are necessary to qualify for a CI; however, these levels are continually changing as both hearing aid and cochlear implant technology advances. The age at which the hearing loss occurred and whether it occurred before (prelingual) or after (postlingual) the acquisition of spoken language are important factors in assessing the potential success of a CI. Children and adults with postlingual deafness derive benefit from cochlear implantation. In children, there is rapid improvement in the first 6 months after implantation with continued improvement beyond 2 years, whereas in adults improvement usually plateaus during the second year after implantation. Study of children with prelingual deafness indicates that most experience benefit from their implant with regard to speech perception. The younger the age of the child at the time of implantation, the more benefit they obtain, as there is greater plasticity in the auditory system. However, progress can be slow and may not be appreciable for a year or more. Cochlear implantation is typically not performed in adults who are congenitally deaf or lost hearing at an early age. Although the procedure is occasionally performed, the outcome in this group of patients is poor due to prolonged auditory deprivation and presumably auditory neuronal atrophy.

Pathology

In the normal-hearing individual, transduction of sound waves into electrical activity that can be transmitted to the auditory nerve and then onto the brainstem and higher auditory centers occurs via depolarization of hair cells in the organ of Corti. Aging, chronic noise exposure and many disease processes (meningitis, labyrinthitis, viral inner ear infections, autoimmunity, ototoxic drugs, cochlear otosclerosis, and skull base fractures) can lead to the loss of these hair cells. Additionally, the organ of Corti may be absent in many cases of congenital deafness. The cochlear implant assumes the role of transduction, delivering a signal to the auditory nerve that can be transmitted to the auditory cortex.

Treatment

Most surgeons prefer to place the CI in the better hearing ear. A skin flap is made posterior to the ear and a canal wall down mastoidectomy performed. The internal receiver-stimulater component of the CI is placed in a recess created in the skull posterior and superior to the mastoidectomy. The facial recess is opened and a cochleostomy is made anterior to the round window into the basal turn of the cochlea to allow for placement of the electrode in the cochlea. More extensive surgery is required if the cochlea is obstructed or obliterated. A transmitter, held in place by a magnet, a microphone, and a speech processor are worn externally. Generally the skin flap is allowed to heal for 4 to 6 weeks before the external devices are fitted and activated.

Imaging Findings

CT

Computed tomography (CT) has been the main imaging modality in the preoperative assessment of CI candidates. Cochlear aplasia and absence of the cochlear nerve are absolute contraindications to cochlear implantation. Absence of the cochlea is readily apparent on CT. Absence of the vestibulocochlear nerve is suggested on CT if the diameter of the internal auditory canal (IAC) is less than 2.5 mm; however, the cochlear nerve may be absent even if the IAC is normal. The cochlear nerve canal can also be assessed on CT, with the assumption that a normal canal will only be formed in the presence of a normal cochlear nerve. A cochlear canal less than 1.4 mm in diameter suggests the possibility of a cochlear nerve abnormality.

In patients with less severe cochlear abnormalities, cochlear implantation can usually be performed. This includes cochlear hypoplasia, Mondini malformation, enlarged vestibular aqueduct, and incomplete partition of the cochlea. However, surgery may be complicated in these cases by perilymph oozing or gushing.

Labyrinthine ossification can result from meningitis, otitis media, otosclerosis, trauma, or labyrinthectomy. Cochlear implantation can be performed in the presence of cochlear ossification, although the surgery is more challenging. Thus cochlear ossification and its extent should be noted on preoperative CT. Fibrous obliteration of the cochlea is more accurately detected on T2-weighted magnetic resonance imaging (MRI) as opposed to CT.

Other abnormalities of the temporal bone are important to note on CT, as they may affect the surgical approach. These include a hypoplastic mastoid process, dense mastoid sclerosis, facial nerve dehiscence, aberrant facial nerve course, aberrant carotid artery, persistent stapedial artery, or protruding jugular bulb. Evidence of acute otitis media should be noted and treated prior to surgery to prevent meningitis or labyrinthitis.

Postoperatively, temporal bone radiographs can demonstrate the position and integrity of the implant as well as determine the depth of insertion of the electrode array. If radiographs cannot determine the position of the implant, CT can demonstrate whether it is intra- or extracochlear. The electrode normally is advanced into the cochlea 20 to 24 mm or for approximately one and a half turns. On CT the electrode tip should extend into the middle turn of the cochlea. On plain radiographs the actual number of electrodes entering the cochlea can be counted. This is important clinically as auditory performance after CI may be a function of electrode insertion depth. CT is also the study of choice in evaluating postoperative infection, especially for detecting fluid collections below the receiver/stimulator (**Fig. 51–1, Fig. 51–2, Fig. 51–3,** and **Fig. 51–4**).

MRI

Preoperative MRI assessment is best accomplished with heavily T2-weighted sequences, which provide optimal contrast between nerves and cerebrospinal fluid and between the membranous and bony labyrinth. Hypoplasia or absence of the cochlear nerve can be visualized, particularly on sagittal images through the IAC. Cochlear obliteration due to fibrosis can be identified as loss of the normal high signal in this structure on the T2-weighted images.

A CI has generally been considered a contraindication to MRI, as the implant may heat, induce a current, or become dislodged. More recent studies have suggested that MRI at 1 to 1.5 tesla may be safely

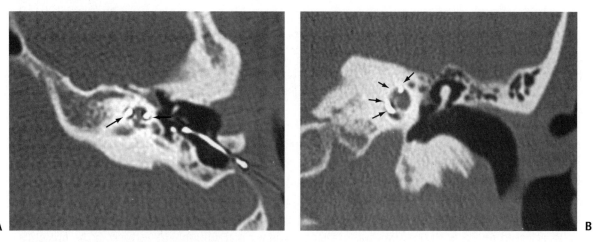

Figure 51–1 Axial **(A)** and coronal **(B)** computed tomography (CT) shows the normal position of the electrodes situated in the middle and basal turns of the cochlea (*arrows*).

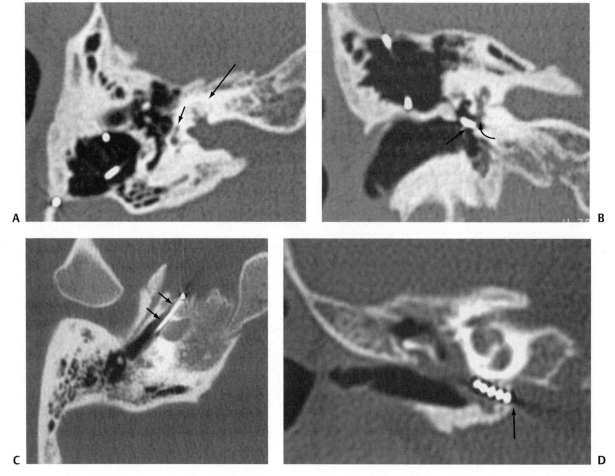

Figure 51–2 Malposition of the cochlear electrode. **(A)** The electrode was unable to be passed through the cochlea secondary to advanced labyrinthitis ossificans. Note the advanced ossification of the cochlea (*large arrow*) and vestibule (*small arrow*). **(B)** The electrode tip (*straight arrow*) has been misplaced in the middle ear cavity just inferior to a narrowed round window (*curved arrow*). **(C)** In a different patient, the electrode has been misplaced through the eustachian tube (*arrows*). **(D)** In another patient, the electrode has been placed underneath the cochlea and is abutting the carotid canal (*arrow*).

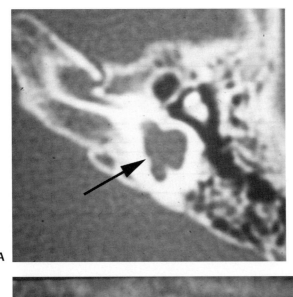

A

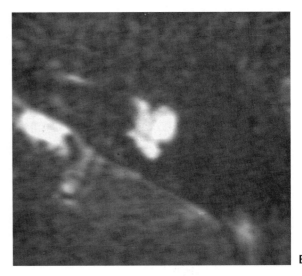

B

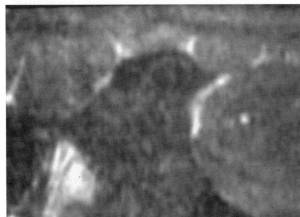

C

Figure 51–3 **(A)** Axial CT demonstrates a common cavity malformation (*arrow*). **(B)** Axial and **(C)** sagittal constructive interference in a steady state (CISS) (7 mm) show absence of the internal auditory canal, indicating cochlear nerve aplasia. This is a contraindication to cochlear implantation.

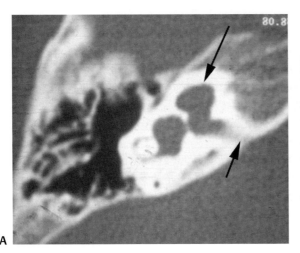

A

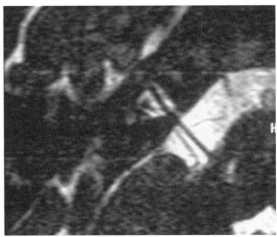

B

Figure 51–4 **(A)** Axial CT shows cochlear hypoplasia (large arrow) and stenosis of the IAC (*small arrow*). **(B)** Axial CISS (7 mm) shows the cochlear nerve to be present (*arrows*).

Based on these findings, this patient underwent a cochlear implant.

performed in patients with a CI. However, each patient should be assessed individually as to the risks versus benefits of the MRI examination.

IMAGING PEARLS _____

• CT is the primary imaging modality in the preoperative assessment of CI candidates.
• MRI may be helpful preoperatively in assessing the presence or absence of the cochlear nerve and in detecting labyrinthine fibrosis.
• Postoperatively the majority of CIs can be accurately evaluated with plain films. CT should be reserved for patients with an abnormal electrode course seen on plain films or patients with malfunctioning electrodes.

Suggested Readings

Baumgartner WD, Youssefzadeh S, Hamzavi J. Clinical application of magnetic resonance imaging in 30 cochlear implant candidates. Otol Neurotol 2001;22:818–822

Bettman R, Beek E, Van Olphen A. MRI verses CT in assessment of cochlear patency in cochlear implant candidates. Acta Otolaryngol 2004;124:577–581

Gantz BJ, Perry BP, Rubinstein JT. Cochlear implants. In: Canalis RF, Lambert PR, eds. The Ear: Comprehensive Otology. Philadelphia: Lippincott Williams & Wilkins, 2000:633–645

Gleeson TG, Lacy PD, Bresnihan M. High resolution computed tomography and magnetic resonance imaging in the pre-operative assessment of cochlear implant candidates. J Laryngol Otol 2003;117:692–695

Hughes GB, Pensak ML, eds. Clinical Otology, 2nd ed. New York: Thieme, 1997:395–405

Jain R, Mukherji SK. Cochlear implant failure: imaging evaluation of the electrode course. Clin Radiol 2003;58:288–293

Lo WWM. Imaging of cochlear and auditory brain stem implantation. AJNR Am J Neuroradiol 1998;19:1147–1154

Miyamoto RT, Robbins AM, Kirk KI, et al. Aural rehabilitation. In: Hughes GB, Pensak ML, eds.: Clinical Otology, 2nd ed. New York, NY: Thieme Medical Publishers, Inc. 1997; 395–405

Ramsden RT. Cochlear implants and brainstem implants. Br Med Bull 2002;63:183–193

Shpizner BA, Holliday RA, Roland JT. Postoperative imaging of the multichannel cochlear implant. AJNR Am J Neuroradiol 1995;16:1517–1524

Stjernholm C, Muren C. Dimensions of the cochlear nerve canal: A radioanatomic investigation. Acta Otolaryngol 2002;122:43–48

Teissl C, Kremser C, Hochmair ES. Magnetic resonance imaging and cochlear implants: Compatibility and safety aspects. J Magn Reson Imaging 1999;9:26–38

White RJ, Lane JI, Driscoll CL, et al. Pediatric and adult cochlear implantation. Radiographics 2003;23:1185–1200

CHAPTER 52 Otosclerosis

Ellen G. Hoeffner

Epidemiology

Genetic, viral, and immunologic factors have been implicated in the etiology of otosclerosis. Studies of familial otosclerosis indicate autosomal dominant transmission with incomplete penetrance. Approximately 60% of patients with otosclerosis have a family history of the disease. Some research points to the measles virus as a possible etiologic agent, with clinical disease developing in those with a persistent measles virus infection and a hereditary predisposition. Other studies suggest that autoimmunity may play a role in the development of otosclerosis.

The disease is most common in the white population and rare in the black population. There is a female preponderance, with a female-to-male ratio of 2:1. It has been reported to be more rapidly progressive in females, and symptoms may worsen during pregnancy.

Clinical Features

Progressive hearing loss, conductive, mixed, or sensorineural, over the course of many years is the primary clinical symptom. Eighty percent of cases are bilateral with onset of hearing loss occurring at ages 15 to 45 years. With fenestral otosclerosis, hearing loss is generally conductive, with the otosclerotic plaque impinging of the anterior crus of the stapes, resulting in mechanical stiffness and ultimately fixation. Cochlear otosclerosis usually occurs in conjunction with fenestral disease, and the hearing loss is usually mixed. Rarely, patients may have isolated cochlear otosclerosis and a purely sensorineural hearing loss. Up to 75% of patients may have tinnitus and 25% vestibular symptoms. Otoscopic examination typically reveals a normal tympanic membrane, although 10% of patients may have a reddish hue behind the tympanic membrane, termed Schwartze sign. This sign is related to increased vascularity of the otic capsule in active cochlear otosclerosis.

Pathology

Embryologically, the otic capsule develops from mesenchymal tissue with a cartilaginous framework present at approximately 8 weeks of gestation and enchondral ossification beginning at approximately 16 weeks. Calcification of the otic capsule is complete by 1 year of age. After this, there is normally little bone remodeling and no osteoclastic or osteoblastic activity in the otic capsule. In the early stage of otosclerosis there is pathologic resorption of the enchondral bone of the otic capsule by osteoclasts and vascular proliferation, a process referred to as otospongiosis. In the late stage of disease there is deposition of new bone by osteoblasts, resulting in formation of dense sclerotic bone. Usually the two stages coexist. The result is areas of disorganized bone that do not follow the normal contours of the otic capsule. This abnormal bone can extend into the middle ear or the perilymphatic spaces.

Fenestral otosclerosis involves the bone just anterior to the oval window, a location corresponding to the embryologic fissula ante fenestram. The otosclerotic plaque impinges on the anterior crus of the stapes, resulting in mechanical stiffness and conductive hearing loss. With progression of disease, complete fixation of the stapediovestibular articulation or replacement of the oval window by otosclerotic bone may occur. Progressive disease may extend posteriorly along the oval window to involve the fossula post fenestram. Cochlear (retrofenestral) otosclerosis involves the bone surrounding the cochlea. It is hypothesized that diffusion of cytotoxic enzymes from the otosclerotic foci into the cochlear fluid produces the sensorineural hearing loss. Cochlear otosclerosis is rarely isolated and is usually associated with fenestral otosclerosis.

Treatment

Treatment of the conductive hearing loss is primarily surgical. The exact surgical procedure is based on the extent of disease and may vary from stapes mobilization, partial stapedectomy, stapedotomy, to complete stapedectomy and prosthesis placement.

Retrofenestral otosclerosis has in the past been a relative contraindication to cochlear implantation. However, patients with profound sensorineural hearing loss from otosclerosis have generally shown benefit from cochlear implantation, although there are special technical considerations in this patient population. Otosclerosis may result in obliteration of the round window and ossification of the cochlea, which may necessitate drill-out of the basal turn of the cochlea or insertion of the electrode array into the scala vestibule rather than the scala tympani. These patients may also have a higher incidence of incomplete electrode insertion and facial nerve stimulation.

Medical treatment consists of sodium fluoride, vitamin D, and calcium carbonate. Approximately 30% of patients treated in this manner improve and 50% show no worsening of symptoms.

Imaging Findings

CT

Otosclerosis is best diagnosed by thin-section computed tomography (CT) (1 mm or less). Overlapping sections should be used to decrease volume-averaging effects. Otosclerotic bone is usually more lucent than the normal bone of the otic capsule, but can be sclerotic. Sclerotic bone is thought to represent a more mature or inactive form of the disease.

Fenestral otosclerosis refers to disease involving the lateral wall of the labyrinth. The most common location of fenestral disease is just anterior to the oval window, with this area being affected in 75 to 95% of cases. This is typically seen as an area of demineralization along the anterior oval window. With disease progression the abnormal new bone may enlarge and protrude into the middle ear cavity, narrow the oval window, or thicken the stapes footplate. According to a study by Veillon et al, a stapes footplate greater than 6 mm should be considered pathologic. Rarely, the otosclerotic foci will be dense, with bone thickening being the main radiologic finding. Fenestral disease can also affect other areas along the lateral wall of the labyrinth, including the round window, cochlear promontory, and tympanic segment of the facial nerve canal.

Cochlear otosclerosis is identified as demineralization around the cochlea on CT. The rim of demineralization may nearly completely surround the cochlea, referred to as the double ring or fourth turn sign. Demineralization may abut the lumen of the labyrinth or be separated from it by denser bone. CT findings of fenestral otosclerosis are usually present. In the chronic, sclerotic phase, remineralization can occur and the CT may appear normal. The differential diagnosis of cochlear otosclerosis includes osteogenesis imperfecta, Paget disease, ankylosing rheumatoid arthritis, and syphilis.

Computed tomography is also necessary in the pre- and postoperative assessment of patients with otosclerosis. In patients with fenestral otosclerosis who are potential stapedectomy candidates, the facial nerve canal, round window, ossicular chain, vestibular aqueduct, and jugular foramen should be evaluated. Facial nerve dehiscence with impingement of the facial nerve on the oval window should be noted prior to placement of stapes prosthesis. Round window obliteration by otosclerotic foci generally portends a poor result if prosthetic stapedectomy is performed. Ossicular chain deformity should be noted.

Computed tomography can also be used in the postoperative assessment following prosthetic stapedectomy or cochlear implantation (**Fig. 52–1, Fig. 52–2,** and **Fig. 52–3**).

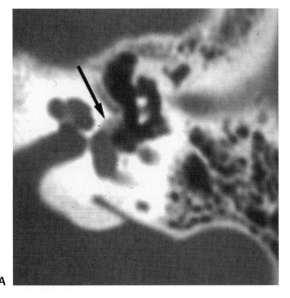

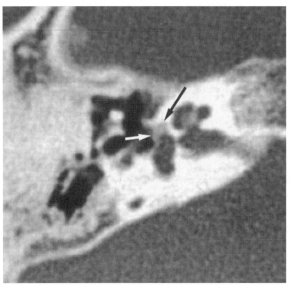

A   **B**

Figure 52–1 Fenestral otosclerosis. **(A)** Axial image demonstrating an otosclerotic focus as an area of lucency just anterior to the oval window (*arrow*), corresponding to the location of the fissula ante fenestram. **(B)** Axial image in a different patient showing lucent otosclerotic focus anterior to oval window (*black arrow*) with bone enlargement protruding into middle ear (*white arrow*).

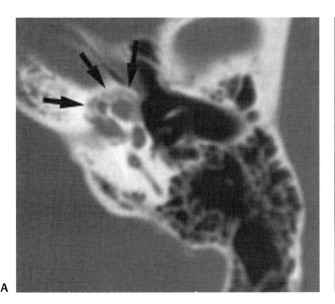

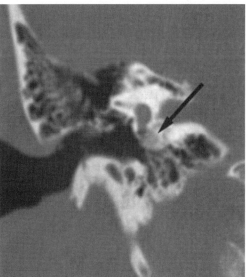

A   **B**

Figure 52–2 Cochlear (retrofenestral) otosclerosis. **(A)** Axial CT image showing cochlear otosclerosis with rim of lucency around the cochlea (*arrows*). **(B)** Coronal CT image with otosclerotic focus adjacent to and impinging on the round window (*arrow*).

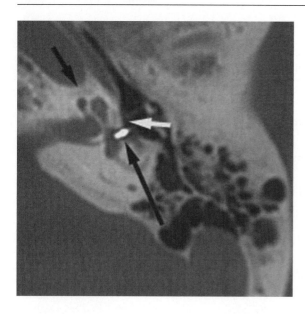

Figure 52–3 Fenestral and cochlear otosclerosis with stapes prosthesis. Axial CT image in a patient with fenestral (*white arrow*) and cochlear otosclerosis (*short black arrow*). A stapes prosthesis is present (*long black arrow*).

MRI

Magnetic resonance imaging (MRI) may be helpful in assessing the activity of cochlear otosclerosis. The demineralized bone surrounding the cochlea enhances on T1-weighted images in the active phase of the disease, presumably due to contrast pooling in the vascularized otospongiotic bone. Subtle increased signal may also be seen surrounding the cochlea, or the cochlea may be indistinct on T1-weighted images without contrast.

Magnetic resonance imaging with T2-weighted images may be helpful in ensuring there is normal fluid in the membranous labyrinth in potential cochlear implant candidates. Loss of the fluid signal indicates fibrosis or bone formation within the labyrinth.

If a patient does require MRI for evaluation of otosclerosis following the placement of a stapes prosthesis, the safety of imaging such a patient with an implant that may be ferromagnetic or rendered ferromagnetic by the manufacturing process is a primary concern. The concern is that the electromagnetic fields generated by MRI scanners may cause movement or heating of the prosthesis. Most ossicular prostheses have not displayed ferromagnetism when tested with a 1.5-tesla (T) static magnet, though there have been a few exceptions. One stapedectomy piston prosthesis made of ferromagnetic stainless steel was grossly displaced by the MRI scanner; this prosthesis was later recalled, and patients that had the prosthesis implanted before the recall were given MRI safety warning cards. More recently, several stapes prostheses made of nonferromagnetic material showed gross movement when placed in a 1.5-T scanner. The authors theorized that the manufacturing process induced the ferromagnetism and suggested testing every stapes prosthesis for movement, by placing the prosthesis in a sterile Petri dish and using a handheld sterile magnet, prior to implantation.

With the advent of higher field strength clinical magnets, studies performed on middle ear prostheses have shown that multiple prostheses made of nonferromagnetic stainless steel do show displacement when tested ex vivo at 3-T field strength or higher, even though these same prostheses may have shown no movement in MRI scanners of 1.5-T field strength or lower. The clinical significance of ex vivo movement of prostheses is uncertain; when implanted in cadaveric temporal bones or animal models, these prostheses remained in proper position, without demonstrable movement or damage to the oval window, even at field strengths of 3 T or higher. Prostheses made of metals such as titanium, platinum, nickel, or nitinol are presumably safe in the MRI environment, as these are nonferromagnetic and cannot acquire ferromagnetic properties through the manufacturing process.

IMAGING PEARLS _____

- Thin, overlapping section CT is the primary imaging modality used to diagnose fenestral and cochlear otosclerosis. MRI may play a small role in determining the activity of cochlear otosclerosis.
- The most common abnormality in fenestral disease is demineralization anterior to the oval window.
- A rim of demineralization surrounding the cochlea is the most common finding in cochlear disease. The differential diagnosis includes osteogenesis imperfecta, Paget disease, ankylosing rheumatoid arthritis, and syphilis.

Suggested Readings

Chole RA, McKenna M. Basic science review pathophysiology of otosclerosis. Otol Neurotol 2001;22:249–257

Niedermeyer HP, Arnold W. Etiopathogenesis of Otosclerosis. ORL J Otorhinolaryngol Relat Spec 2002;64:114–119

Roland PS, Meyerhoff WL. Otosclerosis. In: Bailey BJ, ed. Head and Neck Surgery—Otolaryngology, 2nd ed. Philadelphia: Lippincott-Raven, 1998:2083–2096

Rotteveel LJC, Proops DW, Ramsden RT. Cochlear implantation in 53 patients with otosclerosis: demographics, computed tomographic scanning, surgery and complications. Otol Neurotol 2004;25:943–952

Ruckenstein MJ, Rafter KO, Montes M. Management of far advanced otosclerosis in the era of cochlear implantation. Otol Neurotol 2001;22:471–474

Saki O, Curtain HD, Hasso AN, et al. Otosclerosis and dysplasias of the temporal bone. In: Som PM, Curtin HD, eds. Head and Neck Imaging, 4th ed. St. Louis: Mosby, 2003

Schwartz JM. The otodystrophies: diagnosis and differential diagnosis. Semin Ultrasound CT MR 2004;25:305–318

Veillon F, Riehm S, Emachescu B. Imaging of the windows of the temporal bone. Semin Ultrasound CT MR 2001;22:271–280

Vicente Ade O, Yamashita HK, Albernaz PLM. Computed tomography in the diagnosis of otosclerosis. Otolaryngol Head Neck Surg 2006;134:685–692

CHAPTER 53 Fibrous Dysplasia

Vaishali Phalke

Epidemiology

Fibrous dysplasia (FD) is a disease that commonly affects adolescents and young adults. There are two major forms of disease: monostotic FD, which involves a single bone, and polyostotic FD, which involves multiple bones. Monostotic FD is most common in adults younger than 30 years of age (75%); 10% of patients with monostotic FD have temporal bone involvement.

Polyostotic FD affects young children, with the skull and face being more commonly involved (50%). It accounts for 25 to 27% of all FD cases, and involves two or more osseous sites generally on the same side. Most patients present at a young age usually with craniofacial asymmetry. A subtype, McCune-Albright syndrome, is defined by a clinical triad of polyostotic FD, which is usually unilateral, endocrine dysfunction, and café-au-lait spots. This subtype accounts for 3 to 5% of all FD cases and affects more bones more severely at an earlier age. It primarily occurs in females. Fibrous dysplasia (monostotic and polyostotic) is thought to arise from sporadic gene mutation.

Clinical Features

Craniofacial lesions are more frequently polyostotic, and affect the skull and face in 40 to 60% of cases, whereas monostotic FD affects the skull and face in 25%. The most common clinical presentation is conductive hearing loss. Occasionally patients may present with tinnitus, dizziness, pain, trismus, and multiple cranial neuropathies due to involvement of the middle and posterior cranial fossa. Patients may also complain of swelling, pain, and tenderness.

Pathology

Gross specimens have variable consistency, which may range from soft-rubbery to gritty-firm. There is progressive replacement of bone by abnormal proliferative fibrous tissue intermixed with poorly formed and irregularly arranged trabeculae of woven bone, and thus on histologic examination the lesion shows fibrous tissue with intramural bone trabeculae. The lesions originate in the medullary cavity and expand outward toward the surrounding cortical bone. Normal bone is replaced by an irregular array of spindle-shaped mesenchymal cells resembling fibroblasts. These benign-appearing cells form whorled patterns and poorly formed bony trabeculae, gradually causing expansion, distortion, and weakness of the bone with a normal, but thinned cortex remaining in place. These expansile lesions can compress surrounding structures such as cranial nerves.

Treatment

The treatment is usually conservative management. Radiation therapy is thought to increase the likelihood of malignant transformation.

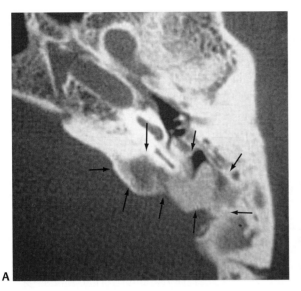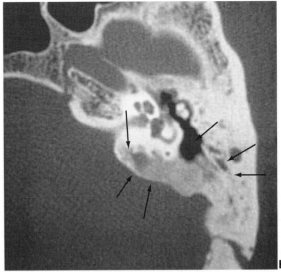

Figure 53–1 (A,B) Axial CT obtained through the temporal bone demonstrates a focal area that has the typical ground-glass appearance of fibrous dysplasia (*arrows*).

Imaging Findings

CT

Computed tomography (CT) demonstrates an expansile bone lesion with a surrounding rind of sclerotic bone. Different patterns of craniofacial FD involvement have been described: pagetoid, sclerotic, and cystic. The cystic form (with an incidence of 21%) is hypodense except along its edges; the pagetoid form (with an incidence of 56%) has a ground-glass appearance; and the sclerotic form (with an incidence of 23%) has a uniform density approaching that of cortical bone. Stenotic narrowing of the external auditory canal may also be present (**Fig. 53–1**).

MRI

On magnetic resonance imaging (MRI), FD presents as an expansile bone lesion hypointense on both T1- and T2-weighted images. Depending on the amount of bony trabeculae, cellularity, and cystic and hemorrhagic changes, the signal intensity may vary on T2-weighted imaging and lesions may be hyperintense. Most lesions generally show enhancement on T1-weighted images on administration of gadolinium either centrally or peripherally. MRI can be useful to evaluate soft tissue structures adjacent to the lesion, especially the cranial nerves.

Bone scan may be performed; it is nonspecific but sensitive in evaluation of skeletal lesions in cases of polyostotic FD. There is increased radionuclide accumulation in the perfusion and delayed bone phase.

IMAGING PEARLS

- The bony lesion on CT shows a ground-glass matrix with disease activity relating to CT appearance, with the cystic form likely representing the most active and the sclerotic form representing the least active form of the disease.
- Other differential diagnostic considerations include ossifying fibroma, giant cell tumor, osteoblastoma, and intraosseous meningioma.

Suggested Readings

Brown EW, Megerian CA, McKenna MJ. Fibrous dysplasia of the temporal bone: imaging findings. AJR Am J Roentgenol 1995;164:679–682

Casselman JW, De Jonge I, Neyt L. MRI in craniofacial fibrous dysplasia. Neuroradiology 1993;35:234–237

Hullar TE, Lustig LR. Paget's disease and fibrous dysplasia. Otolaryngol Clin North Am 2003;36:707–732

Jee WH, Choi KH, Choe BY. Fibrous dysplasia: MR imaging characteristics with radiopathologic correlation. AJR Am J Roentgenol 1996;167:1523–1527

Lustig LR, Holliday MJ, McCarthy EF. Fibrous dysplasia involving the skull base and temporal bone. Arch Otolaryngol Head Neck Surg 2001;127:1239–1247

Papadakis CE, Skoulakis CE, Prokopakis EP. Fibrous dysplasia of the temporal bone: report of a case and review of its characteristics. Ear Nose Throat J 2000;79:52–57

Ringel MD, Schwindinger WF, Levine MA. Clinical implications of genetic defects in G proteins. The molecular basis of McCune-Albright syndrome and Albright hereditary osteodystrophy. Medicine (Baltimore) 1996;75:171–184

Weinstein LS, Chen M, Liu J. Gs mutations and imprinting defects in human disease. Ann N Y Acad Sci 2002;968:173–197

Yabut SM. Malignant transformation of fibrous dysplasia: a case report and review of the literature. Clin Orthop Relat Res 1988;228:281–289

CHAPTER 54 Paget Disease

Ashok Srinivasan

Epidemiology

Paget disease, also called osteitis deformans, is a chronic disorder that involves approximately 3% of adults above 40 years of age and approximately 10% above 80 years. The etiology is unknown, though it has been attributed to genetic and infectious factors and there is familial and geographic clustering.

Clinical Features

Paget disease may be asymptomatic and detected incidentally or can present with involvement of one or multiple bones. Although Paget disease can involve various portions of the auditory apparatus like the external auditory canal, otic capsule, and petrous pyramid, ossicular involvement is rare. The most common clinical symptom in temporal bone involvement is hearing loss, which can be conductive, sensorineural, or mixed. Other symptoms that can occur include tinnitus and vertigo.

Pathology

Involvement of the temporal bone in Paget disease can be divided into four phases: osteolytic, mixed, osteoblastic, and remodeling. In the initial osteolytic phase, there is increased vascularity and cellularity in the bone marrow. There is active osteoclastic resorption of bony trabeculae with resultant lytic areas, which appear radiolucent. In the intermediate mixed phase, there is replacement of lytic areas by new bone formation that causes an increase in bone density and thickness. The simultaneous lytic and blastic activity can result in a cotton-wool appearance. This phase is followed by an osteoblastic phase, which results in replacement of the medullary cavity by avascular fibrous tissue and formation of lamellar, densely packed bone. The sclerotic form of Paget disease is uncommon in the temporal bones. The inactive osteoblastic bone can undergo remodeling into normal lamellar bone with distinct haversian canals.

Treatment

Treatment consists of symptomatic relief. Salmon calcitonin can promote healing of osteolytic lesions, and stabilize hearing.

Imaging Findings

CT

High-resolution computed tomography (CT) of the temporal bone reveals decreased bone density due to demineralization. In the mixed phase, there can be a heterogeneous appearance of mixed lysis and sclerosis. Bone thickening can also be seen in the mixed and sclerotic phases of the disease. Paget disease typically starts at the petrous apex and progresses inferolaterally. Involvement of the otic capsule is a late manifestation. Paget disease can also affect the footplate of stapes resulting in hearing loss, can involve the mastoid process, and can cause basilar invagination due to softening of the skull base. The

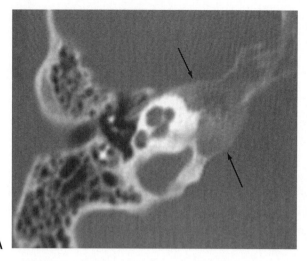

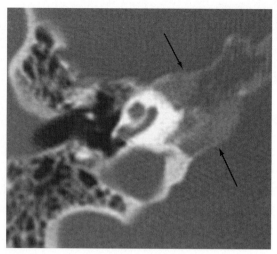

A   B

Figure 54–1 (A,B) Axial images demonstrate demineralization and expansion of the bone involving the petrous apex (*arrows*). The dense bone surrounding the inner ear is not affected, but involvement of this bone may be seen in very advanced cases and is unusual.

eighth cranial nerve can be stretched by the basilar invagination, which can contribute to the hearing loss (**Fig. 54–1**).

MRI

The magnetic resonance (MRI) findings in temporal bone Paget disease are variable depending on the stage of the disease. With marrow replacement by fibrous tissue, there is decreased marrow signal on T1-weighted images. The presence of hemorrhage or slow flow in enlarged vascular channels can result in a patchy, heterogeneous high signal within the bone. In the hypervascular osteolytic and mixed phases of the disease, contrast enhancement has been observed. The increased metabolism and blood flow can also produce diffuse meningeal enhancement.

IMAGING PEARLS _____

- The differential diagnosis includes fibrous dysplasia, hyperparathyroidism, metastatic lesions, pyknodysostosis, and meningiomas.
- The clinical information is key to the differential diagnosis.

Suggested Readings

d'Archambeau O, Parizel PM, Koekelkoren E, Van de Heyning P, De Schepper AM. CT diagnosis and differential diagnosis of otodystrophic lesions of the temporal bone. Eur J Radiol 1990;11:22–30

Ginsberg LE, Elster AD, Moody DM. MRI of Paget disease with temporal bone involvement presenting with sensorineural hearing loss. J Comput Assist Tomogr 1992;16:314–316

Jardin C, Ghenassia M, Vignaud J. Tomographic and CT features of the petrous bone in Lobstein's disease. One case and a review of the literature. J Neuroradiol 1985;12:317–326

Nager GT. Osteitis deformans Paget. In: Nager GT, ed. Pathology of the Ear and Temporal bone. Baltimore: Williams & Wilkins, 1993:1011–1050

Nager GT. Paget's disease of the temporal bone. Ann Otol Rhinol Laryngol 1975;84:1–32

Swartz JD, Vanderslice RB, Korsvik H. High resolution computed tomography: Part 6. Craniofacial Paget's disease and fibrous dysplasia. Head Neck Surg 1985;8:40–47

Whyte MP. Heritable metabolic and dysplastic bone diseases. Endocrinol Metab Clin North Am 1990;19:133–173

CHAPTER 55 Osteogenesis Imperfecta

Ashok Srinivasan

Epidemiology

Osteogenesis imperfecta (OI) is a genetic disorder that results in deficient fibroblastic and osteoblastic activity. This connective tissue disorder is caused by an error in type I collagen with resultant clinical manifestations that affect not only bone formation but also skin, teeth, and other connective tissue. In greater than 90% of cases, OI results from mutation in one of two genes: the *COL1A1* gene on chromosome 17 and the *COL1A2* gene on chromosome 7, which encode the chains of type 1 collagen.

Clinical Features

There are four major types of OI with a variable degree of clinical manifestations. Type I is the most common and mildest form of the four and type II is the most severe form. The typical manifestations are a tendency of bone to fracture with minimal trauma, blue sclerae, and deafness. Other clinical features include faulty dentin production, joint dislocations, easy bruisability, and hyperflexibility. In type II, multiple in utero fractures of the skull, vertebrae, and chest wall may result in death in utero or shortly after birth.

Pathology

Histopathologic examination of specimens removed from OI patients can provide clues to the type of hearing impairment that can be expected in these patients. In type II patients, there is markedly delayed and deficient ossification in the three layers of the otic capsule with microfractures, deformities, and dehiscence involving the otic capsule and middle ear ossicles. Conductive hearing loss in these patients is mainly due to fractures that commonly involve the crus of the stapes or the handle of the malleus. These fractures can lead to discontinuity of the ossicular chain or to fixation, by ankylosis, of the head of the malleus to the medial attic wall. Adult-onset hearing loss with OI, therefore, can be a conductive type and is not always progressive.

Reports of type I, though scant, have shown extensive bony labyrinth involvement by the otosclerotic or spongiotic foci that can affect all parts of the otic capsule, including the vestibules and semicircular canals. Also otosclerosis can be found concurrently with OI infrequently, and hearing loss can be due to otosclerosis, OI, or both. Conductive hearing loss is often due to stapedial footplate fixation secondary to otosclerosis, and less frequently, from stapedial crural fracture. Spongiotic involvement of the cochlear capsule and the cochlear promontory, and destruction of cochlear and vestibular endochondral bone can contribute to progressive sensorineural hearing loss.

Treatment

Treatment is essentially supportive, though in some instances stapedectomy may yield good results for conductive hearing loss.

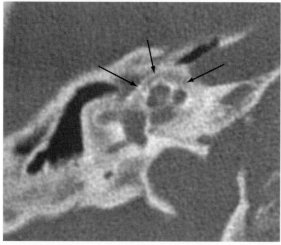

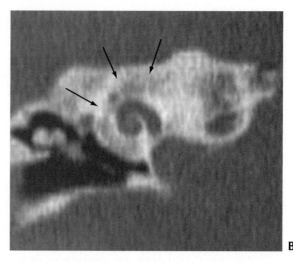

A

B

Figure 55–1 (A) Axial and **(B)** coronal reformations show the typical pericochlear lucencies (*arrows*) that can be seen in patients with OI. These findings are indistinguishable from retrofenestral otosclerosis.
(Courtesy of Regina Lúcia Elia Gomes, MD and Eloisa S. Gebrim, MD)

Imaging Findings

CT

On computed tomography (CT), there is proliferation of undermineralized bone around the otic capsule, which can extend from the labyrinth into the middle ear cavity. Dysplastic bone formation involving the stapedial crura can result in oval window obstruction. The facial nerve can be compressed by narrowing of the facial canal. The demineralization can even reach up to the level of the superior semicircular canal. The differential diagnosis is retrofenestral or cochlear otosclerosis, but OI can be distinguished by more extensive involvement and the clinical history (**Fig. 55–1**).

MRI

The specific inner ear imaging findings of OI have not been well defined. Magnetic resonance imaging (MRI) can be helpful in evaluating the platybasia and basilar invagination that can be seen in patients with OI that result from the "soft bones" (**Fig. 55–2**).

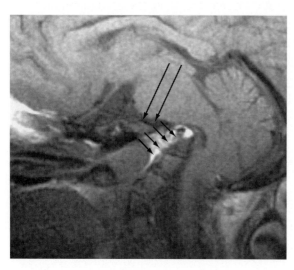

Figure 55–2 Sagittal T1 images obtained through the skull base in a patient with OI shows flattening of the clivus (platybasia) (*long arrows*) and superior displacement of the cervical spine through the foramen magnum (basilar invagination).

IMAGING PEARLS

• Bilateral otic capsule involvement by demineralized bone is typical, due to the systemic nature of the disease.

• The key differential diagnosis is retrofenestral or cochlear otosclerosis. Clinical history and extent of temporal bone involvement are clues toward the diagnosis.

Suggested Readings

Ablin DS. Osteogenesis imperfecta: a review. Can Assoc Radiol J 1998;49:110–123

Berger G, Hawke M, Johnson A, Proops D. Histopathology of the temporal bone in osteogenesis imperfecta congenita: a report of 5 cases. Laryngoscope 1985;95:193–199

Byers PH, Steiner RD. Osteogenesis imperfecta. Annu Rev Med 1992;43:269–282

Garretsen TJ, Cremers CW. Stapes surgery in osteogenesis imperfecta: analysis of postoperative hearing loss. Ann Otol Rhinol Laryngol 1991;100:120–130

Marion MS, Hinojosa R. Osteogenesis imperfecta. Am J Otolaryngol 1993;14:137–138

Nager GT. Osteogenesis imperfecta of the temporal bone and its relation to otosclerosis. Ann Otol Rhinol Laryngol 1988;97:585–593

Sando I, Myers D, Harada T, Hinojosa R, Myers E. Osteogenesis imperfecta tarda and otosclerosis: a temporal bone histopathology report. Ann Otol Rhinol Laryngol 1981;90:199–203

Sykes B, Ogilvie D, Wordsworth P, Anderson, Jones N. Osteogenesis imperfecta is linked to both type I collagen structural genes. Lancet 1986;2:69–72

Sykes B, Ogilvie D, Wordsworth P. Consistent linkage of dominantly inherited osteogenesis imperfecta to the type I collagen loci: COL1A1 and COL1A2. Am J Hum Genet 1990;46:293–307

Tabor EK, Curtin HD, Hirsch BE, May M. Osteogenesis imperfecta tarda: appearance of the temporal bones at CT. Radiology 1990;175:181–183

Zajtchuk JT, Lindsay JR. Osteogenesis imperfecta congenita and tarda: a temporal bone report. Ann Otol Rhinol Laryngol 1975;84:350–358

CHAPTER 56 Lymphoma

Hemant Parmar

Epidemiology

Middle ear malignant tumors are rare. The most common malignant tumors are squamous cell carcinoma and adenocarcinoma. Middle ear lymphoma is an extremely rare tumor with few cases reported in the literature. These include Hodgkin disease, B-cell non-Hodgkin lymphoma, and mycosis fungoides. Most of the cases occur as extension from temporal bone, which is affected in generalized lymphoma or as an extension from the nasopharynx. Primary malignant lymphoma of the middle ear was first described by Malik et al. Lymphoma of the middle ear may arise from the mucosa of the mastoid antrum, tympanum, or tympanic orifice of the eustachian tube, because these regions have a layer of lymphoid tissue deep to the epithelium that can be a primary site for lymphoma. It is also suggested that a small number of circulating lymphocytes home into areas that are usually not regarded as secondary lymphoid tissues.

Clinical Features

Clinical symptoms of middle ear lymphoma are nonspecific. Patients present with ear pain and varying degrees of conduction deafness and facial nerve palsy. Systemic manifestations of lymphoma in the form of fever, lethargy, and weight loss may be present. Some patients have enlarged neck lymph nodes. Initial ear presentation mimics infection; however, symptoms do not respond to medical therapy. Unresponsiveness to medical treatment and development of facial nerve paralysis should alert the clinician to suspect middle ear malignancy like lymphoma.

Pathology

Microscopic examination reveals tissue fragments of heterogeneous population of small degenerated cells, inflammatory cells, and medium to large atypical cells. The atypical cells demonstrate hyperchromatic, convoluted, and clefted to absent amphophilic cytoplasm. Tumorlike necrosis can be also seen. Immunohistochemical staining (including pan-B and pan-T markers) demonstrates strong positive staining of atypical cells with leukocyte common antigen. For immunohistochemical examination, an unfixed specimen is preferable.

Treatment

Uniform therapy for middle ear lymphoma has not been established. Recently it has been shown that for localized intermediate and high-grade non-Hodgkin lymphoma, chemotherapy plus radiotherapy is superior to chemotherapy alone. The value of central nervous system prophylaxis is unknown. Cases have been reported where the facial paresis resolved after appropriate chemotherapeutic treatment.

Imaging Findings

CT

Computed tomography (CT) scan appearances for lymphoma are nonspecific, and tissue biopsy is required for diagnosis. On CT scan, lymphoma is seen as a soft tissue mass in the skull base or middle ear. The surrounding bone may have a permeative appearance. Involvement of the middle ear may result in bulging of the tympanic membrane. In the initial stages there is no bony or ossicular destruction or dehiscence of the facial nerve canal, whereas late stages show permeative destructive lesions (**Fig. 56–1**).

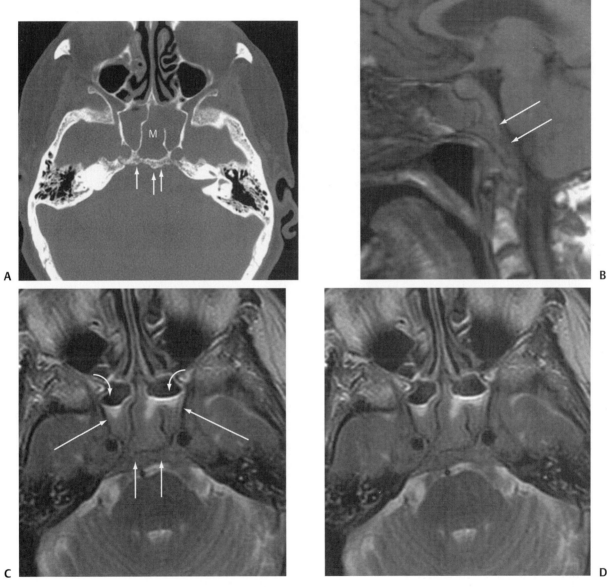

Figure 56–1 Skull base lymphoma. **(A)** Axial computed tomography (CT) of the skull base reconstructed in bone algorithm shows a soft tissue mass involving the sphenoid sinus (M). There is a permeative appearance to the posterior wall of the sphenoid sinus (*arrows*) indicating bone invasion. **(B)** Noncontrast sagittal T1-weighted magnetic resonance image (MRI) obtained in the same patient as in **A** shows replacement of the normal high signal in the clivus by lymphoma, which has an intermediate signal (*arrows*).

(C) Axial T2-weighted image shows mixed signal within the sphenoid sinus. The central high signal (*curved arrows*) is due to retained secretions. The peripheral intermediate signal in the sinus (*long straight arrows*) is due to lymphomatous involvement. Note the intermediate signal that is located in the prepontine cistern (*short straight arrows*). **(D)** The axial T1-weighted image shows the lymphoma in the sphenoid sinus and prepontine cistern to be an intermediate signal. *(Continued)*

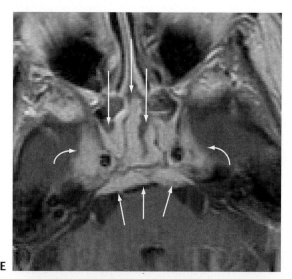

E

Figure 56–1 *(Continued)* **(E)** There is diffuse enhancement of the lymphoma involving the sphenoid sinus (*long straight arrows*), cavernous sinus (*curved arrows*), and prepontine cistern (*short straight arrows*).

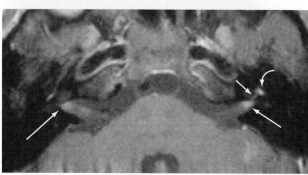

Figure 56–2 Axial postcontrast T1-weighted image with fat suppression shows enhancement of the distal canalicular portion of the internal auditory canal (*long straight arrows*) due to lymphomatous meningitis. There is also enhancement of the left labyrinthine segment of the facial nerve (*small straight arrow*) and the geniculate ganglion (*curved arrow*).

MRI

Magnetic resonance imaging (MRI) is complementary to CT scan, especially to define the disease extent. Like round cell tumors elsewhere, lymphoma shows as an intermediate signal on T1- and T2-weighted images with contrast enhancement. Postcontrast T1-weighted images with fat saturation may help improve the conspicuity of enhancement. MRI also has a role in differentiating tumor from areas of inflammatory mucosal changes, which are hyperintense on T2-weighted images (**Fig. 56–2**).

IMAGING PEARLS

- Lymphomatous involvement of the skull base and temporal bone is a rare tumor.
- The imaging findings are nonspecific, The differential diagnosis should include other neoplastic and inflammatory processes such as Wegener's, sarcoidosis, and fungal diseases, especially if the patient is immunocompromised.

Suggested Readings

Gordin A, Ben-Arieh Y, Goldenberg D, Golz A. Extension of nasopharyngeal to the middle and external ear. Ann Otol Rhinol Laryngol 2003;112:644–646

Kamimura M, Sando I, Balaban CD, Haginomori SI. Mucosa-associated lymphoid tissue in middle ear and Eustachian tube. Ann Otol Rhinol Laryngol 2001;110:243–247

Malik MK, Gupta RK, Samuel KC. Primary lymphoma of middle ear—a case report. Indian J Cancer 1976;13:188–189

Merkus P, Copper MP, Van Oers MH, Schouwenburg PF. Lymphoma in the ear. ORL J Otorhinolaryngol Relat Spec 2000;62:274–277

Scott SN, Burgess RC, Weber PC, Gantz BJ. Non-Hodgkin's lymphoma of the middle ear cleft. Otolaryngol Head Neck Surg 1997;117:S203–S205

Tucci DL, Lambert PR, Innes DJ Jr. Primary lymphoma of the temporal bone. Arch Otolaryngol Head Neck Surg 1992;118:83–85

Suresh K. Mukherji

Epidemiology

Superior semicircular canal (SSCC) dehiscence is the absence of the bony roof of the superior semicircular canal that normally forms the arcuate eminence of the temporal bone **(Fig. 57–1).** The disorder

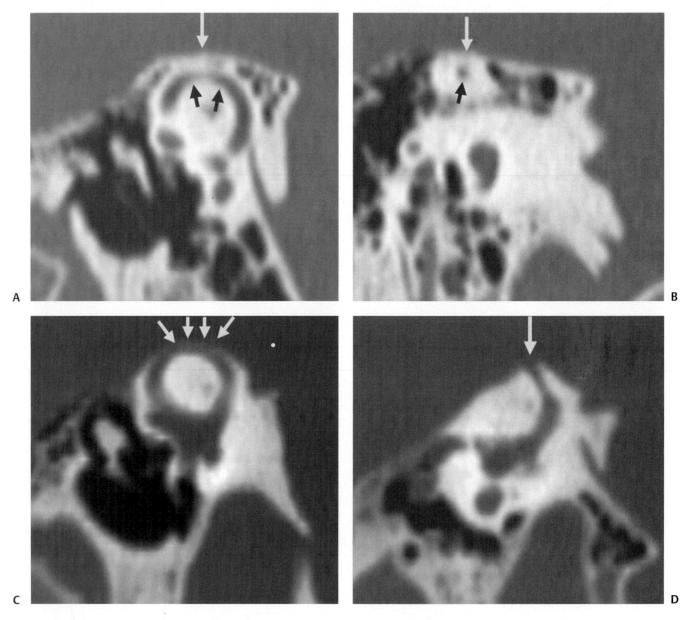

Figure 57–1 Multiplanar reformations obtained en face **(A)** and orthogonal **(B)** to the plane of the superior semicircular canal demonstrates the normal appearance of the canal *(short arrows)* and the bony covering comprising the roof *(long arrows)*. **(C,D)** Absence of the bony roof *(arrows)* indicating dehiscence of the canal.

208

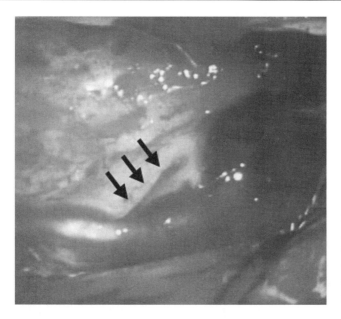

Figure 57–2 Intraoperative photo shows the appearance of a dehiscent superior semicircular canal. Note the linear bony defect in the bone *(arrows)* represents the lumen of the superior semicircular canal, which is visualized due to the roof being absent. (Courtesy of Steve Telian, MD.)

appears to be more common in men (2:1) with a mean age of 42 years. Unilateral involvement is more common, with ~20% patients having bilateral dehiscence of the SSCC.

Clinical Features

Patients with dehiscence of the SSCC present with sound- or pressure-induced vertigo **(Fig. 57–2)**. Patients may present with vertigo or oscillopsia (apparent motion of objects that are known to be stationary) evoked by loud noises (Tullio phenomenon). These findings may also occur by stimuli that result in changes in middle ear or intracranial pressure (pressure on tragus or Valsalva maneuver). The Tullio phenomenon is the classic symptom complex associated with SSCC dehiscence. However, this symptom complex can be seen in other disorders affecting the vestibular system such as perilymph fistula, vestibular migraines, and autoimmune inner ear diseases.

Pathology

The absence of the bony roof functionally results in a "third mobile window" (in addition to the oval and round windows) into the inner ear. As a consequence of the dehiscence, endolymph fluid motion is induced by sound and pressure stimuli, which is the pathogenesis of the typical clinical findings.

Treatment

Accurate diagnosis is essential, as the surgical treatment is quite aggressive and complex. Adequate exposure can only be obtained by a middle fossa approach. There are two primary techniques for repair. One is to place a plug composed of fascia and bone dust and occlude the lumen of the superior semicircular canal. This plug is then covered by fascia and a bone graft. The second option is to preserve the lumen of the SSCC and reconstruct just the roof using fascia and bone graft.

Imaging Findings

CT

Computed tomography (CT) is the modality of choice for imaging patients suspected of having this disorder. The imaging findings are absence of bone forming the roof of the superior surface of the SSCC.

The diagnosis requires submillimeter imaging with multiplanar reformations in planes parallel (in plane) and orthogonal to the course of the SSCC.

MR

Magnetic resonance (MR) can potentially be performed; however, there are possible drawbacks. The bony roof of the SSCC is normally very thin and it may be difficult to characterize this with MR. It is unclear if the in-plane and soft tissue resolution will be superior to that of CT. This may improve with newer sequences that permit submillimeter isovoxel acquisition such as FIESTA, CISS, and VISTA.

IMAGING PEARLS _____

- Optimal CT technique is crucial to detect this abnormality. We recommend contiguous submillimeter acquisition with a slice thickness not to exceed 0.625 mm. Multiplanar reformats in the proper planes (see above) are essential for proper diagnosis.
- We routinely image and reformat both temporal bones, as it is often difficult to locate the proper side based on the clinical findings.

Suggested Readings

Belden CJ, Weg N, Minor LB, Zinreich SJ. CT evaluation of bone dehiscence of the superior semicircular canal as a cause of sound- and/or pressure-induced vertigo. Radiology 2003;226:337–343

Minor LB. Superior canal dehiscence syndrome. Am J Otol 2000;21:9–19

Ostrowski VB, Byskosh A, Hain TC. Tullio phenomena with dehiscence of the superior semicircular canal. Otol Neurotol 2001;22:61–65

INDEX

Note: Page numbers followed by *f* and *t* indicate figures and tables, respectively.